Change Your
Magnetism

Change Your
Life

Change Your
Magnetism

Change Your
Life

How to Eliminate Self-Defeating
Patterns and Attract *True* Success

Naidhruva Rush

crystal clarity **publishers**

Printed in the United States of America

ISBN-13: 978-1-56589-307-8
Epub ISBN-13: 978-1-56589-563-8

1 3 5 7 9 10 8 6 4 2

Cover designed with love by Amala Cathleen Elliott.
Interior design by David Jensen.

Library of Congress Cataloging-in-Publication Data

Names: Rush, Naidhruva, author.
Title: Change your magnetism, change your life : how to eliminate
   self-defeating patterns and attract true success / Naidhruva Rush.
Description: 1st Edition. | Nevada City, California : Crystal Clarity
   Publishers, 2016.
Identifiers: LCCN 2016005741 (print) | LCCN 2016031210 (ebook) | ISBN
9781565893078 (quality pbk. : alk. paper) | ISBN 9781565895638 (ePub)
Subjects: LCSH: Self-actualization (Psychology) | Energy psychology.
Classification: LCC BF637.S4 .R857 2016 (print) | LCC BF637.S4 (ebook)
| DDC
   158.1–dc23
LC record available at https://lccn.loc.gov/2016005741

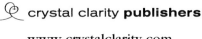 crystal clarity **publishers**
www.crystalclarity.com
clarity@crystalclarity.com
800-424-1055

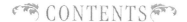 CONTENTS

ACKNOWLEDGEMENTS

I am deeply grateful to Jyotish and Devi Novak, Spiritual Directors of Ananda Worldwide, for encouraging me to write this book. Both Anandi Cornell and James Van Cleave offered suggestions that greatly contributed to the finished product. My sincere thanks also go to Richard Salva of Crystal Clarity Publishers, a superb editor.

I would also like to thank my son, Joseph, whose personal example of strong positive magnetism often came to mind when I was writing these pages. Finally, I owe a huge debt of gratitude to Ananda's founder, Swami Kriyananda, whose lectures and writings on the subject of magnetism transformed my life.

Success in every area of life depends on the power of one's magnetism to attract it. Broadly defined, magnetism is the power of attraction. Ordinary bar magnets attract metal objects according to the power of the magnets. The stronger the magnet, the stronger the magnetism. Magnetism is not only a property of certain metals, however. Applied to people, magnetism is an inner force which attracts people, things, and opportunities that are on the same "wavelength."

A basic principle of magnetism is "like attracts like." We become like the people with whom we mingle, not through their conversation, but through the magnetic vibrations emanating from their bodies and their beings. The person whose magnetism is stronger gives his vibrations to the other.

There are as many different types of magnetism as there are people. Musicians have one kind of magnetism, financiers another, and scientists still another. We must first decide what kind of magnetism we want and then associate with those people who possess it. If we want to become artists, we should associate with talented artists. If we want to become good at business, we should associate with successful business people or leaders. If we want to become strong spiritually, we should associate with devotees of God.

Paramhansa Yogananda—the great spiritual teacher and author of the classic *Autobiography of a Yogi*—described spiritual magnetism as the "power of all powers," and often counseled people, even those seeking material success, to concentrate *first* on developing spiritual magnetism. He said: "Develop power to attract the highest thing, then you can easily attract all lesser things." When we have strong spiritual magnetism, we are able to attract *whatever* else we need: inspiration, money, the right job, a good living situation, or a compatible life partner.

The strength and quality of your magnetism

In the following pages you will find a discussion of magnetism tailored to the needs of people actively seeking a better way to live in today's tumultuous times.

For the sake of clarity, the different aspects of magnetism are often presented as individual and separate, though in actuality they blend together in an inseparable whole. Some aspects of magnetism are foundational. Much like the foundation of a house, they form the supporting structure. To eliminate any one of them is to weaken or collapse the entire structure. Will power, energy, concentration, and enthusiasm fall into this category. These four aspects determine the overall *strength* of your magnetism.

The nine other aspects of magnetism discussed in these pages, starting with the chapter on kindness, determine the *quality* of your magnetism and are what distinguish the sinner from the saint, the mafia capo from a Padre Pio, the corporate defrauder from a Mother Teresa. These nine interrelated aspects might be compared to the brightly colored pieces of glass in a kaleidoscope which, when shaken, form interesting and sometimes beautiful patterns. If you are seeking a more fulfilling life, the challenge is to make choices that will cause the kaleidoscope of your magnetism to resolve into vibrant, divinely attuned patterns.

It is my sincere wish that the following discussion of the thirteen aspects of magnetism will enable you to select choices that lead to true happiness.

PART ONE

THE STRENGTH OF YOUR ENERGY FLOW

1. Will Power And Energy

2. Concentration

3. Enthusiasm

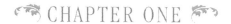

CHAPTER ONE

WILL POWER AND ENERGY

Strong will power is a prerequisite for strong magnetism and for every kind of success. History is full of instructive examples of the life-changing power of will. An especially inspiring example is that of Helen Keller, who was deprived of sight and hearing following a mysterious illness when she was nineteen months old.

Helen Keller: Will power equal to every challenge

Helen Keller was six years old in 1887 when Anne Sullivan, a teacher trained in teaching the blind, entered her life. By then her parents were desperate. Helen was given to tantrums and violent outbursts and had become completely unmanageable.

After winning Helen's confidence, Anne began the process of teaching her. Anne introduced Helen to the world of language and communication by using finger movements to spell words in Helen's hand. An eager and inquisitive student, Helen learned thirty words the very first day. Thereafter, it was Helen who usually led her teacher by the hand as she moved from object to object in her environment, determined to learn the names of familiar objects. From then on, Anne Sullivan was Helen's constant companion.

Throughout Helen's long life, her will power proved equal to whatever challenges she embraced, including obtaining a college education. In 1890, after attending schools for the blind and deaf, Helen gained admittance to Radcliffe College in Cambridge, Massachusetts. She was eighteen years old.

Despite Helen's enthusiasm and determination to work hard, she found the educational process unusually laborious. Anne had to spell all lectures into Helen's hand. Books had to be translated into Braille. Tests were especially difficult: Anne could not be present and directions were sometimes unclear. Nonetheless, in 1904, Helen became the first blind-deaf person to graduate from college, earning her Radcliffe degree *cum laude*. Before graduation, with the help of a Harvard student, Helen wrote her first book, *The Story of My Life*. Thirteen more books would follow. She also became proficient in Latin, Greek, German, and French.

Determined to communicate with others as conventionally as possible, Helen learned to speak and spent much of her life giving lectures. In 1918, at age thirty-one, she began her lifelong work of improving the quality of life for people who were blind or, as she was, both blind and deaf. A tireless advocate, Helen traveled to thirty-nine countries and, through her speeches and personal example, sparked a movement that resulted in the introduction of numerous programs to educate and train the blind and the deaf-blind.

Helen Keller's strong will power was the decisive factor in her being able to attract success in ways considered impossible for a person with her physical handicaps. Other aspects of magnetism were also at work, including enthusiasm and a positive attitude, qualities which we will discuss in later chapters. For Helen, however, will power that translated into perseverance and persistence was clearly the crucial element. In Helen Keller's long life, no obstacle proved too great, no challenge too difficult for her indomitable will power.

Strong will power creates a magnetic field that can attract to us whatever we are seeking. What Helen Keller attracted included a college education; opportunities to improve the lives of people who were deaf or blind and deaf; a circle of devoted friends and supporters that included Alexander Graham Bell, Samuel Clemens (Mark Twain), and Oliver Wendell Holmes—and a deeply fulfilling life.

The greater the will, the greater the flow of energy

Paramhansa Yogananda's stated principle, "the greater the will, the greater the flow of energy," is the foundation of his teachings on magnetism. A corollary to that fundamental principle is: the stronger the flow of energy, the stronger the magnetism.

Magnetism is best understood by an analogy with electricity. Electricity passing through a wire creates a magnetic field. As more electricity passes through the wire, the magnetic field becomes stronger. A strong flow of electricity creates a strong magnetic field. It is generally understood that living near high voltage power lines can be harmful to health. Using the language of magnetism, we can say that high voltage power lines generate a harmful magnetic field and thus a harmful magnetism.

The human body can also be said to have electric wires: the nerves. Whenever we *will* something to happen, we send out through our nerves rays of energy which create a magnetic field. The stronger our will power, the stronger our magnetic field as correspondingly more energy passes through our nerves. Whether we are speaking of electricity or of the human nervous system, it's the *flow of energy* in our bodies that creates magnetism.

Neither our bodies nor this universe is solid. They are both holding patterns of energy. This fact was scientifically confirmed by Albert Einstein in 1905 when he established that matter itself is a vibration of energy. The question then arises: If by will power alone we can increase the flow of energy in our bodies, what is the source of that energy?

The cosmic source of energy

We all draw revitalizing energy from physical sources such as food, oxygen, and sunshine. However, by strengthening our will power and using it in a more conscious way, we are able to draw an *unlimited* supply of energy from the surrounding cosmic energy. The more will power we direct toward a specific goal, the more *energy* we draw from the cosmic source.

Paramhansa Yogananda created a series of "Energization Exercises" to demonstrate these two principles: 1) that by the conscious use of will power, we can draw unlimited energy into the body from the surrounding cosmic energy, and 2) we can consciously direct that energy to the trillions of cells that make up the human body, strengthening and revitalizing them. The exercises take only twelve to fifteen minutes to finish and are marvelously revitalizing to one's body and spirit.*

---

* Contact Ananda via ananda.org for more information.

The daily practice of these exercises trains us to generate and apply energy at the command of our will. Strong will power is the secret to drawing an unlimited supply of energy from the cosmic source. The stronger our will power, the more energy we have to achieve our goals. Summing up: the greater the will, the greater the flow of energy. The greater the flow of energy, the stronger the magnetism.

When our will power is strong, we are able to generate the energy and magnetism needed to accomplish our goals.

Unwillingness: the main obstruction to strong will power

For most people, the word "will" suggests tension and mental strain. "Willingness" more accurately captures the meaning of Paramhansa Yogananda's statement, "the greater the will, the greater the flow of energy." Whenever we truly *want* to do something, there is no resistance or strain. The willingness to perform actions is *always* accompanied by fresh supplies of energy and can produce remarkable feats of strength, as when (to mention only one example) a distraught parent manages to lift a car off of an injured child.

A more familiar example is that of a man (Tom) who, tired and irritable after a challenging day in the office, comes home and flops on the couch. Using the remote control, he turns on the TV and vows not to move again until he is "good and ready." Five minutes later, the phone rings. The caller is an old friend (Bob) who is unexpectedly in town and invites him to dinner and a new play that Tom has wanted to see. Agreeing to meet Bob in thirty minutes, Tom showers, gets dressed, and heads out eagerly to join his friend. After the play, the two of them go to a bistro and talk until well past midnight.

How do we account for Tom's sudden burst of energy? Willingness! The willingness to perform whatever tasks life presents is *always* accompanied by fresh supplies of energy. Mental unwillingness to perform whatever task lies before us is *always* accompanied by a lack of energy. Saying "I can't" or "I won't" to life's challenges, verbally or otherwise, obstructs the energy flow.

Unwillingness is the main obstacle to developing strong will power. Often there is a subconscious resistance, born of fear or laziness, to exercising our will power to the fullest. To achieve our goals, like Helen Keller, we must be completely willing in everything we do. Willingness generates energy and magnetism, which attract the support of cosmic forces in our efforts to achieve success.

Viktor Frankl: indomitable will power

The failure to maintain strong will power often stems from not knowing how to persevere when faced with obstacles or setbacks. Success requires that we be able to exercise our will power to the utmost even in the most dismal of circumstances.

In his book *Man's Search for Meaning*, Viktor Frankl writes that, during his time in a World War II German concentration camp, only his strong will power saved him from what seemed certain death. As a physician and a psychiatrist, Frankl was acutely aware of the great challenge prisoners faced in trying to rise above their physical and mental sufferings. Repeatedly he saw prisoners lose faith in the future and simultaneously lose the will to live.

The crisis usually began in the morning--a prisoner

would refuse to get out of bed and report for inspection. If the prisoner was ill, he would not allow anyone to take him to sickbay. Indifferent to everything around him, the prisoner would lie in his bed, hardly moving, and would soon die.

Frankl writes about the time he too nearly gave up. In constant pain from sores on his feet from having to wear badly worn shoes, each day he had to march a couple of miles to a worksite, every step forward impeded by bitter-cold, winter winds. One day Frankl was on the verge of tears. Hobbling along painfully in a long column of men, weak and thin from insufficient food, he could think only of the cold and pain he was enduring. His mind churned with such thoughts.

At one point he became disgusted with having to think so constantly about comfort and survival. Summoning up all of his reserves, he *willed* his thoughts to turn to another subject. The result was extraordinary. Here is what he writes:

"Suddenly I saw myself standing on a platform of a well-lit, warm and pleasant lecture room. In front of me sat an attentive audience on comfortable upholstered seats. I was giving a lecture on the psychology of the concentration camp! All that oppressed me at that moment became objective, seen and described from the remote viewpoint of science. By this method I succeeded somehow in rising above the situation, above the sufferings of the moment, and I observed them as if they were already of the past. Both I and my troubles became the object of an interesting psychoscientific study undertaken by myself."[*]

Viktor Frankl, through the exercise of strong will power, found a way to raise his energy and transcend the sufferings

---

[*] From *Man's Search for Meaning*.

of the moment. The instant his energy flow became strong, his magnetism shifted and attracted a powerful vision of a future free from the horrors of concentration camp life.

Strong feeling and a powerful will

While we may not find ourselves in a concentration camp, yet, in the relative challenges of everyday life, the same principle applies. Whenever we feel strongly about an endeavor, we can easily summon up the will power and energy needed to achieve our goal. *Feeling*, more than reason, is the motivating force in any endeavor. Feeling, which is centered in the heart, awakens energy. Once that energy is awakened, as it was in Viktor Frankl when he became disgusted with his survival-related thoughts, "will" is the power that directs the energy.

Strong feeling expressed through a powerful will can achieve outstanding success in anything one attempts. The example of Viktor Frankl shows that, once our hearts are engaged, we have an unlimited amount of will and energy at our disposal to call upon whenever needed. Deep, heartfelt conviction gives us the will power and energy to confront our challenges, the courage to remain calm and focused no matter how many difficulties arise, and the determination to bring the assignment to a successful conclusion.

Paramhansa Yogananda writes that "a strong will by its dynamic force creates a way for its fulfillment." When one's will is backed by unflagging courage and faith, it develops into a dynamic power that attracts to itself the desired object or goal. Will power is one of the most important qualities we can train ourselves to develop—to enable us to keep going whether we like it or not. A trait all successful people have in common is that they cannot imagine giving up. If one approach does not work they will try another, and if not that, then still another. They will keep on trying until they find something that works. What stands out most in nearly all success stories is the extraordinary will power required.

The examples of Helen Keller and Victor Frankl also show that calmness and self-control are essential aspects of strong will power. The *will* does not become *will power* until it is directed calmly and with control. Calmness gives us a sense of proportion and renders us less vulnerable to wrong impulses. We will have strong will power when calmly, without mental strain, we are able to control our behavior and focus our full attention on our goal.

Abilities develop with practice.

Many people think, "But I've got to save my strength." It is important, of course, to exercise reason and discretion and to rest periodically as needed. We should not exert our will power to the point that we create such inner tension and mental resistance that our will power flags. Always remember, however, that abilities develop only with practice. Helen Keller's extraordinary life shows that the more we *use* our energy, the more we *generate* energy. As our energy increases, so also does our will power. There is virtually no limit to how much we can accomplish once we set foot *willingly* on the path to success.

It has been said that "will power governs the universe." When one's will is backed by unflagging courage and faith, it develops into a dynamic power that attracts to itself the desired object or goal.

Four ways to strengthen your will power and energy

1. *Develop the habit of perseverance.*

You can strengthen your will power by setting realistic goals for yourself each day and then meeting those goals. Without specific goals, it's much more difficult to develop a habit of perseverance, and without a habit of perseverance, you will not have strong will power. Begin by doing something you always thought you could not do. Don't take on too big a task at the start, but make up your mind to do it.

People fail only because they give up. Do one thing after another that you thought you couldn't do, and you will soon see your life change for the better. Helpful goals include getting up and going to bed at the right times, being punctual for all engagements, and honoring all commitments, even if difficult.

2. *Banish fear and self-doubt.*

There are two things that create a flow of energy. One is will power; the other is clearing the channels for that flow by removing any obstructions. The most common obstruction to strong will power is fear of failure. People are often pulled in two directions at once. So much of their energy is consumed by fear of failing that they do not use their will power strongly enough to succeed.

It's important not to dwell on difficulties. The right approach is to think positively, to believe that you have the ability to achieve your constructive goals, and then to put your full energy into *everything* you do. Don't let the thought of failure enter your mind. No matter what challenges come, continue on step by step with unswerving determination.

3. *See obstacles as opportunities.*

In life obstacles are inevitable. Obstacles challenge us to summon up more energy; without them, we would become lethargic. Try to *welcome* any difficulties you encounter. Each time you face a test courageously, your strength and will power increase. If you do your best in the present, the future will take care of itself. Even if karmic obstacles impede your success, doing your best will speed the dissolution of these and other obstructions. (The impact of karmic obstacles is discussed in chapter 10.)

4. *Think more in terms of energy.*

Energy has its own intelligence, and responds willingly to proper guidance. It can make things happen for you that you yourself could never have planned. To attract abundance in your life, see money as a flow of *energy*, not as a static quantity. See life in the same way—as a flowing river, not as fixed patterns of behavior. When you feel tired, instead of letting down and thinking how tired you are, concentrate on the energy flowing in your body and renewing your strength. The following easy-to-do exercises are very helpful in raising your level of energy.

Exercises* to Increase Your Energy Flow

Whenever you need a boost, repeat each of the six exercises three to five times.

1: Walk vigorously in place while affirming,

I am awake and ready! I am awake and ready!

* These "Superconscious Living Exercises" were created by Swami Kriyananda

2: Extend your arms vigorously out to the side, then in front, then high above the head, affirming, "I am positive! energetic! enthusiastic!" (Before each new movement bring the hands back to the chest.)

I am positive! *(Arms to the side)*

Energetic! *(Arms to the front)*

Enthusiastic! *(Arms high above the head)*

3: Rap your knuckles lightly on the forearms and upper arms, first with the right fist, then with the left, affirming,

I am master of my body! I am master of myself!

4: Rub lightly your arms, legs, hips, chest, and other parts of the body, affirming,

Awake! Rejoice, my body cells!

5: Rap your scalp lightly with your knuckles, affirming,

Be glad, my brain! Be wise and strong!

6: Massage your scalp lightly with your fingertips, affirming,

Awake, my sleeping children! Awake!

Finally, relax your arms at your sides. If needed or desired, repeat the entire series of exercises.

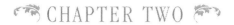

CHAPTER TWO

CONCENTRATION

No effective action can be performed without concentration. Concentration is the ability to withdraw the mind from objects of distraction and place it on one thing at a time. Concentration is essential to the development of will power and magnetism. For our will to become will *power* we must be able to focus and direct our will calmly, with control. When we can withdraw our attention from all diverting objects and focus it one-pointedly on a goal, we are well on the way to developing strong magnetism.

Although the average person is restless, there are times when most people can concentrate very well. Whenever we are truly interested in something, we can easily forget everything else. Our mind and attention are completely focused. While watching a good movie, for example, our concentration is engrossed in whatever is taking place on the screen. Interest, therefore, is an important key to strengthening one's ability to concentrate. Indeed, the following example suggests that the term "interest" can be expanded to include *any* strong motivation.

Kamila Sidiqui: Intensely focused concentration

The *Dressmaker of Khair Khana*, by Gayle Tzemach

Lemmon, is the story of how a group of young women managed to survive after the Taliban took control of Afghanistan from 1999 to 2001. Nineteen-year-old Kamila Sidiqui, one of nine children and the second oldest, was attending college when the Taliban issued an edict stating that 1) women were not permitted to work or attend school, 2) they must remain at home, and 3) whenever in public, they must wear the *chadri*, a shapeless head-to-toe covering with a narrow slit for the eyes.

After Kamila's father, brother, and later, her mother were forced to leave the country to escape imprisonment or death, Kamila, as the oldest sibling at home, needed to devise a plan that would enable her and her seven younger siblings to survive while staying within the Taliban's rules. Although the local economy was collapsing, the market for clothing remained strong; Kamila decided to become a seamstress. Wearing the required *chadri*, she went to the home of her older married sister, an expert seamstress, and asked to be taught how to sew.

During three hours of intensely focused concentration, Kamila learned everything she needed to know: how to thread the sewing machine, move the pedal, and make a simple dress with beading. This dress she would use as a sample to get orders from shopkeepers. Kamila knew that her careful attention to detail would win the respect of shopkeepers, and would thus lead to orders.

In the marketplace, Kamila was always accompanied by the required male escort, in this instance, her thirteen-year-old brother. Conversations with male shopkeepers were always brief and hurried—they would be severely punished by the Taliban if seen talking to a woman. Unable to write anything down, Kamila concentrated one-pointedly on their words and gestures and remembered everything, even changes requested in the patterns for the garments ordered.

Kamila's professionalism and keen attention to detail soon magnetized the steady flow of work that enabled her and many others to survive. As her dressmaking business flourished, Kamila was able to hire and train women outside her family circle, many of whom also worked in their own homes.

Does concentration require mental effort?

Many people assume that concentration requires mental effort, but, in fact, any kind of tension, mental or physical, is an obstacle to developing strong powers of concentration. Deep concentration can only occur when one is deeply relaxed, as when watching an enjoyable movie.

Regular meditation is very helpful for developing the relaxed concentration that translates into the magnetism to attract what we need. Meditation is also an excellent aid in developing mental clarity. If at all possible, one should meditate at least fifteen minutes a day, gradually increasing that time at a comfortable pace, incorporating longer periods whenever possible.

Paramhansa Yogananda recommended that his followers engage in the spiritual exercise known as "japa," the inward repetition of a name of the Divine or of a devotional phrase, a practice which also increases one's powers of concentration. The goal of japa is to live in the constant awareness of God's inner presence. It has been said that when one practices japa successfully, all other considerations melt away "like morning mist before the rising sun." Such, indeed, was the experience of Frank Laubach.

"Worries have faded away."

Frank Laubach: vibrant with joy

Frank Laubach was a Christian missionary who served in the Philippines in the early 1900s. Profoundly dissatisfied with his spiritual life, and inspired by the examples of Christian mystics such as Thomas à Kempis and Brother Lawrence, Laubach determined to try to live every minute of the day with his mind concentrated on God. In *Letters by a Modern Mystic*, a compilation of excerpts from letters written to his father during this time, Laubach discusses his efforts, challenges, and successes.

Upon waking in the morning, even though it might take a long time, Laubach would not get out of bed until he had attained a state of one-pointed focus on God. Throughout the day, whenever his mind wandered, he resolutely brought it back to its one-pointed focus.

Gradually, Laubach was able to keep his mind concentrated on God for longer and longer periods. The sense of effort lessened, replaced by feelings of peace and contentment. No longer did he worry about things. Tasks he had once found difficult became effortless. Most important of all, every day was vibrant with the joy he found in God's presence. He writes:

"Now I *like* God's presence so much that when for a half hour or so He slips out of mind . . . I feel as though I had lost something very precious in my life."

Laubach's deepest, most heartfelt wish was to share the fruits of his discovery with others and, especially, to inspire them to write about their efforts to hold God "endlessly" in mind during every waking moment. "The results," he writes, "would astound the world."

Laubach, in his practice of concentration, was seeking spiritual, not material success, and he succeeded in his quest. His strong concentration magnetized spiritual experiences that filled him with wonder and love for God and humanity. To Laubach, the very universe had become home, and vibrant with the ecstasy of God.

The practice of concentration in meditation, or through japa, strengthens our concentration in all areas of life. Not only does our concentration become progressively stronger, our minds also become more mentally efficient. We are able to do more quickly what would ordinarily take a much longer time, and we more easily find answers to questions and solutions to everyday problems. However, as we develop increasing mental strength, we need especially to guard the quality of our thoughts, because what we think about might very well come true. A fundamental principle of magnetism is "like attracts like." Strong focused will power attracts to us and to others the objects of our thoughts. Our thoughts should always be kind, helpful, and a blessing to others.

Will power and concentration: one and the same

Returning to the example of Viktor Frankl discussed in chapter 1, we can see that will power and concentration are, in a sense, one and the same. Viktor Frankl, by the force of his strong will power, drew his mind to a one-pointed focus and attracted a life-changing vision. Strong will power and a focused mind go hand in hand.

When we can focus our minds one-pointedly, we are well

on the way to developing a powerful will and the magnetism to attract success. The stronger our one-pointed focus, the stronger our magnetism. Concentration is thus essential to developing the kind of will power that produces strong magnetism. If our energy is scattered and goes out in many different directions, we will have very little magnetism.

History teaches that all successful men and women had strong powers of concentration. They knew how to withdraw their attention from objects of distraction and focus it on a goal. Their strong, one-pointed focus generated the magnetism to attract whatever they needed: inspiration, solutions to problems, deep understanding, or material success.

Five ways to strengthen your concentration

1. *Quiet yourself inwardly.*

To reduce the possibility of self-generated distractions, always try to quiet yourself inwardly before attempting challenging tasks. It is impossible to concentrate effectively when your feelings are restless or in a state of agitation. Several rounds of deep breathing can be very helpful in bringing the mind and feelings under control. A helpful exercise is to breathe in through the nose for a count of six to eight, hold the breath for the same number of counts, and exhale for a count of six to eight.

2. *Never divide your concentration.*

Try never to divide your concentration. Do one thing at a time. For example, do not talk on the phone while driving (even where legal, with a hands-free device). You can always make a note to remind yourself of something you may want to pursue in the future, but if you allow your mind to shift from one thing to another, you will never learn to concentrate deeply.

3. *Concentrate on whatever you do.*

When you are with people, put your mind fully on them, even when in a group. Avoid the habits of absent-mindedness and dullness.

4. *Practice concentration in a suitable environment.*

In practicing concentration, always try to find a suitable environment. Quiet places are more conducive to calm concentration than places with outward activity and noise.

5. *Practice throughout the day.*

Practice focusing your mind one-pointedly during specific periods throughout your day. When you notice your concentration slipping, simply stop and become focused again.

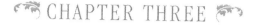

CHAPTER THREE

ENTHUSIASM

Magnetism is the result not only of will power and focused energy but also of *enthusiasm*. For our magnetism to gain power, it is vitally important to summon up strong feeling for what we want to accomplish. Feeling is that capacity of the heart that makes us interested in doing things. Without strong feeling for what we want to accomplish, our magnetism will have little power and we are unlikely to achieve even modest goals.

Enthusiasm is the motive power behind every important achievement, and all true greatness. To care deeply about what we do strengthens our will power and concentration, and gives us the determination to succeed.

Booker T. Washington: Enthusiasm magnetizes success.

Booker T. Washington, one of the early African-American leaders, and the founder of Tuskegee Institute in Alabama, was born into slavery. However, even as a youngster he sought out every opportunity to acquire an education.

After emancipation, Washington's family moved to West Virginia where, at age fourteen, he secured a job in the household of Mrs. Ruffner, a woman from the North who taught him the importance of cleanliness and of doing things promptly. While working for Mrs. Ruffner, Washington was able during certain months to attend school for a few hours a day, but his real goal was to attend the newly established college for blacks in Virginia: Hampton Institute.

Washington arrived in Hampton, Virginia in 1873, hungry, tired, and dirty from sleeping in the open or in wagons. As soon as he reached Hampton Institute, he presented himself to the head teacher for assignment to a class. He had been so long without proper food, a change of clothing, and a bath that the teacher had doubts about admitting him. She did not refuse to admit him, but continued admitting other students while he stood by and waited.

After some hours, the head teacher asked him to take a broom and sweep one of the classrooms. In *Up from Slavery*, Washington writes, "Never did I receive an order with more delight. . . . I had the feeling that in a large measure my future depended upon the impression I made upon the teacher in the cleaning of that room."

Washington approached the task with will power, concentration, and enthusiasm. First he swept the floor three times. Then he dusted it four times with a dusting cloth. After that, he dusted the woodwork, and every bench, table, and desk in the room. In the process, he moved every piece of furniture and thoroughly cleaned every corner of the room, and also every closet. When he was finished, he reported to the head teacher, whom he described as a "'Yankee' woman" who "knew just where to look for dust."

The head teacher inspected the floor and closets, and then took her handkerchief and rubbed it on the woodwork, the table, and the benches. When she was unable to find one bit of dirt on the floor, or a particle of dust on any of the furniture, she quietly remarked, "I guess you will do to enter this institution." Hearing these words, Washington describes himself as "one of the happiest souls on earth."

Enthusiasm and excitement are different.

As eager as Booker T. Washington was to prove himself, his enthusiasm never spilled over into excitement. His feelings were calmly focused as he went about the task of cleaning the room.

For the will to become will *power*, it must be directed calmly, with control.

Excitement stimulates the will. So also does enthusiasm. In both cases, it is the will that generates energy. The energy generated by calm enthusiasm takes us into what yogis teach is our inner center in the spine; the exhilaration of excitement, by contrast, takes the mind outward, away from our inner center, and often leads to errors of judgment and to disappointment.

It has been rightly said that nothing great has ever been accomplished without enthusiasm. Human nature can be divided into two aspects, reason and feeling. Science teaches that the main, if not the only way to arrive at truth, is to exclude feeling altogether. From the life stories of great scientists, however, we learn that they were (and are) men and women of deep feeling, as well as completely dedicated to the search for scientific truth. Without deep feeling and enthusiasm for what they were doing, they could never have made such important discoveries. Thomas Edison is an excellent case in point.

Thomas Edison: "I was never myself discouraged."

The phonograph, Thomas Edison's first original invention, brought him international acclaim. When he was unable to find financial backers to develop the invention, he turned his attention to the development of an incandescent light bulb. His main challenge was to find a durable filament, one which would burn for an extended period in a high-vacuum glass bulb. During the next fourteen months, Edison conducted over forty-three thousand experiments, using every conceivable kind of material. He finally settled on a carbon-based filament that would burn for nearly 1200 hours.

The key to Edison's success was his unflagging energy and enthusiasm in the face of constant difficulties. "The electric light," he said, "has caused me the greatest amount of study and has required the most elaborate experiments. I was never myself discouraged, or inclined to be hopeless of success, but I cannot say the same for all my associates."

Although his associates had pleaded with him, after twenty thousand failures, to give up the attempt, Edison's intuitive certainty of the existence of such a filament fueled his enthusiasm and impelled him to keep on trying until he succeeded.

"Act enthusiastic and you will be enthusiastic."

Dale Carnegie wrote and lectured on the power of enthusiasm, giving illustrations of people who found that, by going through the motions of being enthusiastic, they actually *became* enthusiastic. His formula was: "Act enthusiastic and you will be enthusiastic."

He told an interesting story of a baseball player called

Pep Betgar who had the nickname "Pep" because he was such a fireball of energy. Betgar, however, at the beginning of his career, was so lacking in energy that he was transferred from the major leagues to the minors. Since Betgar did not want to stay in the minor leagues, he decided he would show people that he did, in fact, have energy. He didn't actually *feel* any more energy, but he decided to *act* as if he did. By going through the motions of being energetic and enthusiastic, his will power gradually strengthened and he found that, in fact, he now *had* energy and enthusiasm.

In books and lectures, Dale Carnegie urged people not to wait for circumstances to transform their indifference into enthusiasm. "Even if you feel uninspired," he told his audiences, "act as though you were overflowing with enthusiasm." He cited convincing examples of people who had been failures in life but, by following this principle, in a very short time became outstanding successes. When we act out an attitude, the action itself functions as an affirmation of that attitude.

"The greater the will, the greater the flow of energy." Put another way, if we act as if we have will power—if we go through the motions of being positive, enthusiastic, and energetic—our energy flow becomes stronger. As discussed above, Yogananda taught that the conscious use of will power draws energy into the body from the surrounding cosmic energy. When we act in the manner I've described, we begin to connect with the surrounding cosmic energy and start to draw more and more of that energy into ourselves. Similarly, we can also revitalize ourselves by persistently *thinking* that our body is full of vitality. Whenever we feel physically or mentally weak, we can fill our minds with thoughts of energy and enthusiasm and then visualize that energy and enthusiasm vitalizing all the cells of our bodies.

We can be interested all the time.

Enthusiasm is not conditioned by anything outside ourselves. We don't have to wait until something *interests* us. An effective way of climbing out of the pit of indifference is to express enthusiasm vigorously in both word and action, even if we feel no enthusiasm in our hearts. By focusing our minds with complete enthusiasm on *everything* we do, we can be interested all the time. The example of Booker T. Washington teaches that even the most menial tasks can be done with one-pointed attention and enthusiasm.

If we express enthusiasm in every activity, our will power and concentration will grow very strong. The greater our enthusiasm, the greater our flow of energy and ability to succeed at anything we set out to accomplish. Once we form the habit of enthusiasm, we will find it much easier to persevere in the face of temporary setbacks. Whatever we do, we, like Booker T. Washington, should do it with genuine interest, one-pointed attention, and enthusiasm.

PART TWO

THE QUALITY OF YOUR ENERGY FLOW

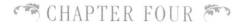

CHAPTER FOUR

KINDNESS

We've been discussing the *strength* of a person's energy flow and the kind of attitudes and practices that create a strong, focused flow of energy—will power, concentration, and enthusiasm. Strong magnetism depends also on the *quality* of our energy, which is determined primarily by our habitual attitudes. Kindness and other positive attitudes are very important for developing strong magnetism. Unkindness, and the disrespect and discourtesy it attracts, will eventually weaken even the strongest magnetism.

Kindness: a selfless energy

True kindness is a loving, selfless, all-giving energy, reflecting a heartfelt concern for the well-being of others. To be truly kind, we must express kindness not only to our family and friends, but to all in need of compassion and encouragement.

Paramhansa Yogananda epitomized such all-giving kindness. Yogananda once went to a cane shop, not because he needed a cane but because canes helped to ground his energy more firmly on the material plane. Being a representative of an organization, he wanted to spend the organization's money wisely, and so he bargained to get the best price he could. When the bargaining was over, Yogananda glanced at his surroundings and thought, "This man has such a poor shop; I want to help him." He then gave the shopkeeper back more money than he had saved through bargaining.

Back at his ashram, Yogananda said, "What a poor floor that man had. I think I'll get him a new carpet." Yogananda, because he lived in the consciousness of seeing God in all beings, was always kind, even to complete strangers. The more strongly grounded we are in a loving, selfless concern for others, the stronger our magnetism to attract to ourselves whatever we truly need.

Kindness as a way of life: The ten Boom family

An especially inspiring account of the magnetic power of kindness is *The Hiding Place*, by Corrie ten Boom. Corrie, a single woman in her fifties, lived in Holland with her watch-maker father and her older sister, Betsy, above her father's Haarlem shop.

After Germany's successful invasion of Holland in 1940, the members of Corrie's extended family became involved in the effort to find safe homes for Jews. Corrie's older brother, a minister, operated a nursing home staffed by young Jewish men disguised as women. Corrie's nephew, the son of her younger sister, was actively involved in the Dutch underground movement, an organized effort to help Jews find secure housing in rural areas outside Haarlem or to escape to a neutral country.

By the summer of 1943, the ten Boom home had become the center of a spreading network of people dedicated to helping Jews in whatever way possible. Corrie, her father, and sister also began sheltering in their home those Jews whose appearance or health made them too great a risk for safe homes outside the city. To create a secret room where the six Jews living in the house could hide in the event of a Nazi raid, a false wall was built in Corrie's bedroom on the top floor of the house.

Inevitably, on February 28, 1944, the raid came. Corrie was ill in bed when the secret alarm sounded. By the time she was dressed, one of the Nazi agents was already in her room, observing every move. Months before, Corrie had packed a small bag to take with her if arrested and jailed. In it were a Bible, clothing, toiletries, vitamins, aspirin, iron pills for her sister Betsie's anemia, and much more. She writes that the bag "had become a kind of talisman for me, a safeguard against the terrors of prison."

Corrie wanted desperately to take the bag with her as she and the guard headed downstairs, but the bag was standing directly in front of the sliding panel leading to the secret room. She knew that by taking it, she would draw the Nazi agent's attention "to the last place on earth" she wanted him to look. She wrote that leaving that bag behind was "the hardest thing I had ever done." By so doing, Corrie demonstrated the selfless, loving concern for others at the heart of true kindness, a concern she would demonstrate repeatedly during and after her imprisonment by the Nazis.

Boundless kindness: "The Lady with the Lamp"

Typical situations for the expression of kindness are interactions involving two or three people. The ten Boom family's assistance to the Jews is an example of kindness on a broader scale involving a number of people acting in a collaborative way. There are times, however, when kindness plays out on a much larger world stage. One inspiring example is the life of Florence Nightingale, whose pioneering efforts brought about worldwide health care reform and magnetized support for nursing as an honorable profession for women of all social classes.

Nightingale was born in 1820 to an elite, affluent British family. At the time, nursing was considered inappropriate for woman of her social class. At age sixteen, she experienced a deep inner call to help the sick and wounded and became convinced that serving in this way was her God-given purpose in life. Nothing could dissuade Nightingale from pursuing her true calling. In1844, despite her parents' objections, she enrolled as a nursing student at the Lutheran Hospital in Kaiserswerth, Germany. This decision marked a major turning point in her life.

Florence Nightingale is possibly best known for the role she played during the Crimean War, a war fought by Great Britain against Russia, chiefly on the Crimean Peninsula. At the time, Nightingale was serving as head of the Institute for the Care of Sick Gentlewomen in London, where she had impressed everyone with her skill, dedication, and humility. After Britain received reports about the deplorable conditions for wounded British soldiers at the main British camp in the Crimea, in October 1854, Nightingale and a team of nurses, many of whom she had trained, were sent to organize the care of wounded soldiers at the British base hospital.

Conditions at the hospital were indeed deplorable: medicines were in short supply; hygiene was grossly neglected, infections were common and often fatal; and adequate food was lacking. Nightingale concluded that most soldiers at the hospital had died not from their wounds but from poor nutrition, lack of supplies, and the overall lack of sanitary conditions.

The efforts of Nightingale and her team of nurses so improved the unsanitary, life-threatening conditions at the British base hospital that the death rate dropped by two-thirds. It was during her service in the Crimea that Florence Nightingale came to be called "The Lady with the Lamp" by soldiers moved by her great compassion. An account appeared in *The Times*:

> She is a "ministering angel" without any exaggeration in these hospitals, and as her slender form glides quietly along each corridor, every poor fellow's face softens with gratitude at the sight of her. When all the medical officers have retired for the night and silence and darkness have settled down upon those miles of prostrate sick, she may be observed alone, with a little lamp in her hand, making her solitary rounds.

Nightingale's experience in the Crimea was a major influence on her later career and the importance she placed on sanitary conditions, not only in hospitals but also in working class homes. Considered the founder of modern nursing, Nightingale combined deep compassion for the ill and wounded with a brilliant mind and a dedication to establishing nursing as an honorable health care profession.

Despite widespread acclaim and recognition, Florence was always humble. Possibly for this reason, upon her death, her relatives declined the offer of burial in Westminster Abbey.

Agape means kindness: Martin Luther King, Jr.

Does the selfless, loving, all-giving energy at the heart of true kindness apply to efforts to bring about change in society as a whole? This was the question Martin Luther King, Jr. sought to answer as a seminary student studying to become a minister. King searched for a way to reconcile what he had read about the power of Christian love with the stark reality that love had not ended slavery in the nineteenth century. Nor had it created an integrated America in the twentieth century. But if love was ineffective as a tool for social change, King wondered, by what means could one reform society?

The answer came when King attended a lecture in which Mahatma Gandhi's teachings on nonviolent resistance were presented. Nonviolent resistance, as taught by Gandhi, was predicated on love for the oppressor and on a belief in divine justice. Gandhi had shown that even if we are violently attacked, we could turn the other cheek and, through our suffering, persuade our adversaries of the superior advantages of love and cooperation. Gandhi's term for this approach was "satyagraha," a philosophy that combined love with nonviolent social protest.

In King's mind, Gandhi had succeeded in making love a powerful force for social change. King understood the love meant by "satyagraha" as identical to the Greek concept of "agape"—an impersonal love for all humanity that enables us to see the neighbor in everyone we meet. Reacting to social injustice with hatred creates bitterness and divisions, but an attitude of agape enables a person to perceive all human life as interrelated, and to respond with love and kindness.

Both Gandhi and King succeeded because their reliance

on the power of love magnetized support and followers for their respective movements that would never have materialized had they relied on violence and hate. Gandhi, the main leader of the twentieth-century Indian independence movement in British-ruled India, employed nonviolent means to lead India to independence. Inspired by Gandhi, King, the pre-eminent civil rights leader in America in the 1960s, successfully used nonviolent means to gain basic rights for disenfranchised black Americans.

You can transform yourself overnight.

The character of Scrooge in Charles Dickens' *A Christmas Carol* is a powerful example of the painful consequences of selfishness. His transformation into a kind, caring friend is equally powerful. It tells the reader that if we make up our minds to be kind, we can transform ourselves overnight.

Unkindness toward others blocks a person's energy flow and eventually weakens even the strongest magnetism. Such an outcome is illustrated dramatically by the downfall of ruthless dictators like Adolf Hitler and Joseph Stalin. It is reflected also in the lives of ordinary people who seek success and worldly influence guided by the principle that "the end justifies the means." Trampling over others to reach their individual pinnacles of success, they either fall short of their goals or, in the end, experience the hollowness of their victories.

The most important reason to treat others with kindness is that, by so doing, we affirm our oneness with the omnipresent love and compassion that manifested the universe and all living creatures. We must not assume, as people often do, that certain individuals or groups are excluded from that divine reality and are therefore unworthy of our love and respect. Everyone is an expression of the Divine in the same way that the gas coming through each jet on a burner, though appearing separate from the gas coming through every other jet, is a manifestation of the unifying gas underneath. To hurt another person is, in a real sense, to hurt ourselves. To whatever extent we hurt others, by unkind thoughts or actions, to that extent we weaken our magnetism.

If you have a tendency to be unkind, make up your mind to change. You can start by speaking sincere, kind words to those to whom you have been harsh or impatient. If unjustly criticized, always respond with genuinely courteous language. If you wish to be kind, you don't need to agree about everything; if you do disagree, always remain calm and courteous. Your calm silence or genuinely kind words will often cause the other person to respond in a more positive way.

While being kind to others, try not to focus on what you will receive in return. Try always to live in the faith that the law of karma guarantees that you will get exactly what is your due, neither more nor less. Keep in mind, however, that the *more* you give generously of yourself—to God, to life, and to other people—the more the karmic law will support you in return, and the more people's attitudes toward you will improve.

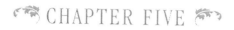

CHAPTER FIVE

POSITIVE ATTITUDES

The cornerstone principle of magnetism is "like attracts like." Our attitudes and expectations of life, whether positive or negative, determine the *quality* of our magnetism. If our thoughts and expectations are positive, we will attract to ourselves success, money, and abundance of every type.

Always pay attention to the slightest hint of negative feelings in your heart. A thought becomes negative and judgmental when there is a negative *feeling* behind it. To help her nuns avoid negative thoughts, St. Teresa of Avila trained them always to think something positive about a person whenever that person came into view. A positive attitude will attract a positive response.

Instead of becoming angry and resentful when something unpleasant comes to you, tell yourself, "Yes, I attracted this energy to myself, and there's something I'm meant to learn from it." Anger and resentment are useless emotions, but you can change things if you say, "It was energy I put out in the past that drew this experience to me. What can I do to prevent this from happening again?"

George Washington crossing the Delaware River: "Victory or death!"

During the Revolutionary War, it was George Washington's positive attitude in the face of great adversity that brought victory to the struggling Continental Army.

In the summer of 1775, Washington was named commander-in-chief of the Continental Army, a position he did not seek. John Adams, who lobbied for Washington's appointment, described Washington as a man of great talents and excellent character who would "unite the colonies better than any other person in the union."

The first eighteen months of Washington's command went badly; he lost battle after battle. By the winter of 1776, many Americans thought it was time to give up. Washington's troops were underfed, poorly armed, and suffering from typhus and dysentery. Unfairly, there was open talk of replacing him. Yet, despite the military losses and public criticism, it was a measure of Washington's character, idealism, and political judgment and that he never lost sight of the need to reverse the tide of defeat. His rallying cry became "Victory or death!"

In an attempt to salvage the war, on Christmas night, 1776, Washington crossed the Delaware River and launched an attack on the British and the Hessians (German soldiers fighting for Britain) in Trenton, New Jersey. Catching them by surprise, the Continental Army took more than nine hundred soldiers prisoner and lost only four men. Washington followed up immediately with another victory at Princeton, New Jersey.

Militarily these were not important victories, but they breathed new life into the revolution. Enlistments poured in from all over the colonies; people everywhere began to feel that it was possible to reverse the course of the war.

Washington, whose very command had been in doubt, now became a national hero. With the aid of France, he achieved final victory in 1783.

Circumstances are neutral.

Your magnetism is defined by your habitual attitudes. Paramhansa Yogananda wrote that "Circumstances are always neutral. Whether they are happy or sad depends entirely upon your state of mind."

If you feel angry, helpless, or discouraged, it is because your own attitudes have attracted these feelings. There is nothing inherently good or bad about any situation. If you have an adequate apartment and a good job, but focus mainly on what is wrong with the apartment and job, those negative attitudes begin to define your magnetism. In a negative state of mind, difficulties become magnified and problems seem insoluble.

When your thoughts are positive, when all of your energy is strongly focused in a positive direction, you will develop the kind of magnetism that attracts inspiration, answers to questions, knowledge—whatever you need. Make it a point to expect the best from life and from other people. Never let fear of failure weaken your will, even if failure is a distinct possibility. A positive attitude enables a person to recover quickly even from great sorrow. The faster the recovery, the greater the spiritual gain.

"Stand up for justice."—Martin Luther King, Jr.

George Washington showed great courage in his decision to launch a surprise attack against the British. Corrie ten Boom and her family were equally courageous in their decision to help the Jews. They knew they would be sent to a concentration camp if their efforts were detected. At a critical point in his work to rid the country of legally enforced racism, Martin Luther King, Jr. found within himself this same level of courage.

King and his associates launched the Montgomery, Alabama bus boycott in 1955 primarily to give blacks the same access to bus seats as whites. A reluctant King was selected as the leader of the effort and thrust into the limelight. Whites determined to maintain the status quo subjected King to psychological warfare.

King began receiving hate letters with threats on his life, as many as thirty to forty a day, and almost as many obscene or threatening phone calls. He had also learned of a plan afoot to assassinate him. Although the boycott and the carpooling effort to get blacks to work were going very well, King found himself wishing for an "honorable way out" of his leadership role in the boycott effort, one that would not injure the cause.

Late one night as he was trying to sleep, King's phone rang with another threatening call: to blow up his house with King and his wife and daughter inside if he did not leave town in three days. King made a cup of coffee and sat down at the kitchen table and prayed. He confessed his weaknesses to God, saying that he was afraid and at the end of his endurance. With head bowed and tears in his eyes, King felt something stirring in himself. It seemed that an inner voice was speaking to him with quiet assurance:

Martin Luther, stand up for righteousness. Stand up for justice. Stand up for truth. And lo, I will be with you unto the end of the world.

King would later affirm that it had been the voice of Jesus telling him to fight on, and that Christ would never abandon him. King now felt stronger. He felt an inner calmness he had never before experienced, and he realized that he could stand up without fear, that he could face *anything*. Whatever happened, God in his wisdom meant it to be.

"Give thanks in all circumstances."

Following their arrest by the Nazis, Corrie and Betsie ten Boom were sent to one of the harshest concentration camps in Germany: Ravensbruck. When they reached the filthy barracks that would be their home, they struggled against nausea at the reeking straw. The place was also infested with fleas. At Corrie's urging, Betsie called on God to show them how they could live in this place, and Betsie found in the Bible they had smuggled into the camp a passage that read: "Give thanks in all circumstances."

Betsie and Corrie thanked God for all the challenging aspects of their living situation, but when Betsie also thanked God for the fleas, Corrie could not find it in her heart to join in Betsie's prayer. A few weeks later, however, she would learn that she and Betsie were able to hold their secret nightly prayer meetings in their barracks only because the guards were so repulsed by the fleas that they refused to enter.

Two choices in every situation

In every situation we can choose to respond negatively or positively. For George Washington, the negative choice would have been to give up, to abandon the revolutionary cause. Instead, he found within himself the courage and optimism to continue. The negative solution for Martin Luther

King, Jr. also was to give up, to surrender to his fears for his own and his family's personal safety, and to reduce his level of involvement in the effort to eliminate a particularly oppressive form of racism.

Sometimes we have to struggle to remain positive. The expression "raise your level of energy" gains new meaning in this context. Washington, King, and the ten Boom sisters found that their challenges demanded of them more effort, and thus more energy. The victory comes when we recommit ourselves to the effort involved and embrace with positive energy whatever circumstances require.

George Washington could have given up. Instead, he went forward. What attitudes enabled him to do this? Courage, optimism, belief in the revolutionary cause, and faith in God. The example of Martin Luther King, Jr. shows that faith in God attracts divine grace, which can give us the strength to face challenges with positive attitudes. It was for this reason that Betsie ten Boom encouraged her sister Corrie to "give thanks in all circumstances." Positive attitudes alone have the magnetic power to attract solutions.

The importance of meditation

In *The New Path,* Swami Kriyananda tells the story of an experience with a negative mood. To overcome it, he sat down and put his full concentration at the point between the eyebrows—what yogis call the "spiritual eye." Focusing at that point created a vortex of magnetism which drew his energy up to the spiritual eye and changed his level of consciousness. Suddenly his mind shifted effortlessly away from the negative mood. He felt wholly positive.

Swami Kriyananda's simple method for banishing negative moods offers powerful encouragement to anyone suddenly caught up in an attitude of negativity. Sit alone in a quiet place. Focus your energy and attention strongly at the point between the eyebrows. Hold that focus until you feel yourself being lifted out of the "fogs of gloom" into an atmosphere of peace, joy, and self-acceptance. We are not our moods or negative energy. The quality of all our characteristics, whether positive or negative, depends entirely on the level of our energy in the *astral spine*—the channel through which bodily energy flows upward and downward, located behind the physical spine. By focusing at the spiritual eye, we can raise our level of energy in a matter of minutes.

Regular meditation is the most effective way of ridding our consciousness of negativity. Affirmations and mental resolutions, though very helpful, are not enough. We also need to introduce a higher dimension of consciousness: superconsciousness.

Through regular meditation we become more centered in the inner Self, and better able to filter out negative thoughts arising from the subconscious mind. It thereby becomes easier for us to direct our will in positive ways. As our will power grows stronger, we can more easily say "no" to whatever we want to exclude from our lives.

Self-expansion: See others as friends.

There are two directions our energy can take: positive or negative. These opposing directions can also be described as expansive or contractive. To help someone in need is a virtue not because scripture or society says so, but for the simple reason that nature implants in us an urge toward self-expansion.

To feel that things are happening *against* us is to feel *contracted*. Similarly, to think, "I'm alone in this universe," is to be contractive. But when we feel that everyone is our friend, we begin to attract people who feel the same way about us.

It is expansive to try to see others as friends, not as rivals or adversaries, whether or not they respond in a positive way. If you find it too difficult to see them as friends, try always to view them with compassion, for they are the ones who suffer most when they express negative attitudes. Even if others, in their ignorance, should hate you, always try to think of them as your brothers or sisters in God.

In all circumstances we have essentially two choices. We can expand our awareness and our feeling of connection to the universe, or we can contract. Often the challenges we face are asking of us that we be a little more expansive—that we include something else in our reality: some other person, some other person's interests, some other possibility. Jesus Christ taught, "It is more blessed to give than to receive." It is more blessed because giving is self-expansive and creates joy in the giver. A self-serving attitude, by contrast, is contractive because it goes against the natural impulse toward self-expansion. By being true to ourselves and a true friend to others, we also gain the friendship of God.

Five ways to banish negative attitudes

1. *Never wish harm to anyone.*

If you are willing, however regretfully, to harm anyone, or to allow harm to befall another, you must pay a price: the loss of your inner peace, happiness, and ability to function at peak efficiency. You will also create in yourself a perception that others are equally willing to harm you, a perception that will lead to inner tension.

2. Devote yourself to right action.

Be as true as possible to right action. Sometimes your intentions are good but your actions are misguided. Even if what you thought was right turns out to be otherwise, God watches your heart, your intentions.

3. Keep your feelings positive.

One of the best ways to generate positive energy is through positive feelings. Negative traits are the consequence of negative currents of energy. Positive feelings alone are capable of directing enough energy to dissolve the vortices of negative traits and draw them upward in a positive flow. A positive attitude demands energy but also uplifts that energy.

4. Choose positive associates.

Associate with people who have a positive outlook, strong will power, and are cheerful in the face of difficulties. More than any other single factor, the company of negative people will cause *you* to become more negative.

5. Gratitude: Thank God for everything.

A key word for developing the right kind of magnetism is gratitude. Gratitude drives out negative feelings—of anxiety, isolation, rejection, and abandonment. You must first actively *feel* grateful and express gratitude consciously. When you open your heart in this way, the negative feelings begin to fade away. An antidote to negative feelings is to make it a habit, several times a day, to thank God for whatever you are experiencing at that moment. Thank Him for the pleasant things, and also for the difficulties. Since we often misjudge what is karmically good or bad, it is best to thank God for everything: good, bad, and indifferent.

Nobility of character

What unites George Washington, Martin Luther King, Jr., and the ten Boom sisters? In the face of circumstances where honorable retreat was possible, where no one would have faulted them had they given up, they remained courageous and steadfast to their commitments. In so doing, they moved beyond positive attitudes to the heights of true nobility.

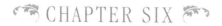

CHAPTER SIX

HONESTY AND TRUTHFULNESS

HONESTY

Honesty and truthfulness, though similar, are different in important respects. Honesty applies primarily to money or other material values. For someone in the business of selling goods or services, honesty means to declare the true value of what one is selling, not to exaggerate its value or fail to disclose known defects.

Honesty also means viewing one's business as a service to others, and not only as a means of earning a livelihood. Thinking of one's business as a service will rule out the likelihood of ever cheating anyone or having any motive other than providing the *best* possible service. Honesty is also the best attitude with which to face unexpected business or other challenges. When we are honest, when we love God and seek His aid, we have the magnetism to attract His help, as illustrated by the following true story.

The lumber company lien: "Show it to me in writing!"

In *A Place Called Ananda,* Swami Kriyananda writes of the time he encountered business dishonesty when the first domes at the Ananda Meditation Retreat were under construction. The foreman of the project had told him the domes would be completed in two weeks. In actuality, the construction took two months. By then, Kriyananda had run out of money.

All of Kriyananda's creditors agreed to partial payments. Even though Kriyananda was making all payments on time, one of his creditors, a local lumber company, put a lien on the Meditation Retreat property. Kriyananda received a letter from the lumber company's attorney threatening to foreclose on the lien if he did not pay within two weeks.

Kriyananda immediately called the lumber company owner, whom he considered a friend, and asked about the lien: Why had he done this when Kriyananda was making timely payments? Possibly sensing an opportunity to seize a valuable piece of property, all the owner would say was, "You see, a person has to be practical." Kriyananda next visited the lumber company's attorney, only to be met with an angry tirade. The attorney shouted, "I don't know anything about an agreement! Show it to me in writing!" Kriyananda and the lumber company owner had a verbal agreement, not a written one.

In the meantime, clinging to his faith in God, Kriyananda gave lectures and programs in the San Francisco Bay Area, doing his best to raise the money to pay the lumber company. Shortly before the two-week deadline, when Kriyananda was giving a program at the home of friends, a young man approached him. He said, "I like what you are doing and would like to make a donation." He wrote a check for three thousand dollars, more than enough to pay the lumber company.

Kriyananda's sincere efforts to pay the debt on time, combined with his faith in God, generated the magnetism to attract that donation.

What does it mean to be honest?

1. Honesty in business means being willing to admit, if asked, that there may be products better suited to a prospective customer's needs than the ones you are selling.

2. If you are the purchaser in a transaction, honesty means not to pretend that the value of what you would like to buy is less than you know or believe it to be.

3. Honesty means not only accepting unexpected business developments but also finding ways to turn them into opportunities for inner growth, such as a suitable occasion to review your priorities.

4. If failure comes, honesty means accepting failure, and not mentally rejecting it, but always trying to make the best of what seems to be bad luck.

5. Perfect *self-honesty*, and the understanding that you alone are responsible for your consciousness, will enable you, in time, to avoid the temptation to blame others for your suffering.

TRUTHFULNESS

Truthfulness is an important aspect of magnetism, but there is considerable confusion over what it means to be truthful. On the level of the divine, absolute truth exists. In this world of relativities, however, there are higher and lower levels of truth. Paramhansa Yogananda offered a few hypothetical situations to illustrate these different levels of truth.

"Suppose," he said, "someone were to approach and ask you to swear on every scripture you considered holy never to repeat what he was going to tell you, and you consented. Suppose he then announced, 'I just put a rattlesnake in So-and-So's bed.' What would you do? Of course you should reveal that secret! Not to do so would be very wrong. And even though it would also be wrong to break your promise, it would be even more wrong to swear to do something without knowing what you were being asked to do."

Higher and lower levels of truth

A further illustration of the different levels of truth appears in *The New Path*. Swami Kriyananda describes a conversation he had with a woman in Czechoslovakia in 1955. She told him of the occasion when Professor Novicky, the leader of a small Self-Realization Fellowship group in Prague, Czechoslovakia, needed to decide in the moment whether a certain person could be trusted:

> [Sometime] after Paramhansa Yogananda's passing, a stranger came to Professor Novicky and requested instruction in yoga. The professor didn't know what to do. Normally he kept his spiritual activities a secret so as not to expose himself to persecution. If this man was a genuine seeker, the professor would want to help him. But if he was a . . . government spy, any admission of interest in yoga might result in a prison sentence . . . .

> [Professor Novicky] prayed for guidance. Suddenly, standing behind the self-proclaimed "devotee," Paramhansa Yogananda appeared. Slowly the Master shook his head, then vanished. Professor Novicky told the man he had come to the wrong place . . . . Sometime later he learned that the man was indeed a government spy.

Kriyananda's informant concluded her story by saying, "I am free to tell this story now, for the good professor died recently, of natural causes."

In *The Hiding Place,* Corrie ten Boom tells of the time her relatives disagreed among themselves on the right course of action regarding truthfulness. At the time, German soldiers occupying Holland were searching homes looking for young men to send to munitions factories in Germany. Corrie's sister Nollie and her husband, Flip, had created an emergency hiding place for their two sons in the potato cellar under the kitchen floor. Covered by a trap door, a large rug, and the kitchen table, it made a suitable hiding place.

Inevitably, the day came when German soldiers burst into Nollie and Flip's house with rifles raised. The entire family was present, including Corrie, Betsie, and their father. Singling out Nollie's terrified fourteen-year-old daughter, Cocky, for questioning, the soldiers demanded to know the exact whereabouts of her two brothers. Cocky replied, "Why they're under the table." As the soldier snatched the cloth from the table, Cocky yielded to a fit of laughter as her bottled-up strain gave way.

"Don't take us for fools," a soldier snapped. He angrily took his leave. Not long after, the home was empty of armsmen.

A somewhat heated family discussion followed. Nollie had trained her children never to lie and supported her daughter, saying, "God honors truth-telling with perfect protection!" Her two brothers, from the vantage point of their hiding place under the table, had their doubts, and so did Corrie.

Going deeply into the subject of truthfulness, Paramhansa Yogananda wrote the following story illustrating the higher and lower levels of truth in a number of different contexts. One of the lessons we can draw from this story is that Cocky's two brothers and her aunt Corrie were right, and that Cocky, out of fear, had chosen a lower level of truth over a higher.

The Saint Who Went to Hades Speaking Truth

One morning, a saint who lived in a forest heard the sound of fast-approaching footsteps. In a few moments a man, his face distorted by fear, halted in front of him. In an imploring voice, he said, "Honored saint, please do not reveal to my pursuing enemies my hiding place in the tree above you, or they will kill me."

The terrified man raced to the top of the tree and hid. The saint had said neither "yea" nor "nay" to the frightened man's request, and the man naturally thought that silence meant consent, and that the saint would not betray him.

As the man lay hidden atop the tree, the saint began to struggle within himself as to what he should do if questioned by this man's enemies. He followed the scriptures strictly and literally. Since the scriptures said not to speak an untruth, and the pursued man would likely be killed if he spoke the truth, he decided to do the following: "If the bandits question me about seeing this man, I shall say, 'I know where he is, but I will not tell you. Do what you like.'"

"You will see Hades for this!"

At last the bandit leader arrived with his retinue. Looking around and seeing only the saint, he asked gruffly if he knew where the man they were seeking was hiding. The saint thought that if he remained silent, the bandit leader would leave. Instead, the bandit leader began to beat him. When severe beatings did no good, the bandit leader brandished his sword, saying, "If you don't answer in five minutes, your body will be headless!"

The saint struggled inwardly regarding what to do. After five minutes he replied, "I know where your man is hiding, but I won't tell you."

The bandit leader then cut off one of the saint's hands. Tauntingly he said, "Tell the truth within five minutes or you will also lose your head!"

Searching for scriptural passages to guide him, the saint remembered one: "Protect your own self above all things. Above all you must achieve your highest ambition of finding God." The saint then pointed to where the doomed man was hiding. Immediately one of the bandits climbed the tree, dragged down the unfortunate man, and hacked him to pieces.

Before the man died, he shouted at the saint, "You will see Hades for this!" The saint, thinking he had done his duty in saving his own greater, more serviceful soul, rejected the dying man's curse as foolish.

Years later, when the saint consciously left his body in the ecstasy of cosmic consciousness, his astral body arrived in the kingdom of heaven. Jama, the keeper of hell, visited him in heaven and told the saint that, before he could take up residence there, he must experience, at least for a time, the loathsome Hades.

The saint replied, "Honored Jama, this is outrageous. I have lived a moral life. I have always followed truth, and performed truthful and just actions. I don't deserve the punishment of visiting Hades, even for a moment."

A truthful action always brings good results.

The great Jama replied, "Honored sir, you are right about everything and correct in all that you did, except for one act. Why were you so foolish as to get your hand cut off, and a man murdered, for stating a *fact*? It seems that you are confused about the difference between a statement of truth and the pronouncement of a fact."

Jama continued: "A just and truthful action always results in good, whereas your statement of a fact, which resulted in great harm to yourself and to that man, was far from ultimate truth. Why didn't you point in the wrong direction in the forest and save yourself from harm, and also save the man's life?

"Even if you had committed the sin of uttering a falsehood, that would have been less sinful than the horrible transgression of being an instrument in the murder of an innocent man. By your silence you let him think you would protect him, and deprived him of the opportunity of seeking another hiding place unknown to you. Then, to save yourself, you betrayed him."

Jama then said, "Honored saint, know that a truthful action always brings good results and is different from a statement of a fact, which may produce good or evil. Always give preference to an action which results in good. To say, 'Hey, Mr. Lame Man,' or 'Hey, Mr. Blind Man,' to a man who is lame or blind may be a statement of fact, but it would be untruthful because not conducive to any good.

"To say, 'Hello, Perfect One,' or 'Greetings, Strong Man,' or 'Hello, Man of Spiritual Vision' may not be statements of fact, but they are wholesome in their effect. Therefore, they are the truth.

"At the same time, remember that it is not good to indulge in cheap lies. Suppose I spied you meditating in your room, and knocked on your door and inquired, 'Mr. Saint, what were you doing?' If you replied, 'I was eating bananas,' you would have sacrificed my trust by lying to be modest. If you had answered my question with, 'Well, I was a little busy,' I couldn't accuse you of lying, nor could I blame you for that evasion.

"Honored saint, one should avoid cheap prevarication, for by this habit you lose the trust of everyone. One may distort facts only when it is a question of life and death, and an unjustly accused person can be saved. One should develop the habit of speaking the truth without unnecessarily advertising all one's secrets. For if you tell your weaknesses to false friends, they will poke fun at you whenever the occasion arises."

In conclusion, the great Jama declared, "Avoid repeating unpleasant facts. Always speak and act in a way that will bring lasting happiness to yourself and others."

Lasting success depends upon right action.

If we are strictly truthful in thought and speech our words will develop the magnetism to become, as Paramhansa Yogananda put it, "binding on the universe." We are all integral parts of the vast web of life. When we speak the truth, we will find support for our statements from the universe itself, and with that support, we will find that everything will always turn out for the best. Without that support, sooner or later things will fall apart. We may, for example, lose friends and find ourselves with little support at critical times.

Truthfulness means much more than adhering to the facts. It means attunement with a higher reality, the one ocean of wisdom underlying all reality. By attunement with that ocean of wisdom we ourselves become wise. We begin to see things as they really are. We understand new or obscure subjects more easily. We find new solutions to problems. And we find new and better ways of achieving our goals.

Determine to live by truth, no matter how difficult. The cost of being true to our word will be light compared to the long-term suffering brought about by dishonesty and untruthfulness. Lasting success of any kind depends upon right action. Even the willingness to indulge in a wrong act occasionally will lead, in the end, to failure or a complete loss of self-worth. The worst failure of all would be the loss of our own integrity.

What is perfect self-honesty?

Although the words honesty and truthfulness are often used interchangeably, in reality there is an important difference. One sees this overlap in discussions of self-honesty. Self-honesty means not to hide from unpleasant facts about ourselves. The more we succeed in accepting ourselves as we are, and in facing our faults and weaknesses for what they are, the easier it will be for us to transcend them.

Often people will say, "I know I've got this problem, but it's okay. I don't have to deal with it." We are living in an age when moral standards are less strict. For spiritual seekers, it's important to remember to go within and ask ourselves whether what we are doing is right or wrong. If we are honest with ourselves, we will rarely go wrong and, if we do, we will quickly correct ourselves. Sincere remorse for past wrong actions is needed before a person can go forward and make the kind of effort needed to advance spiritually, a truth illustrated by the following story.

The woman of Samaria: A lost disciple

Jesus went alone to Samaria, sat on Jacob's well, and asked a low-caste woman to give him a drink from the jug she was filling with water. Yogananda taught that the woman of Samaria was a lost disciple of Jesus from a former incarnation whom he had come to reclaim by awakening her dormant memory of the past.

Before openly declaring himself to be her spiritual teacher, Jesus wanted to test the character of his fallen disciple to see if she could be helped. The woman of Samaria had had five husbands and was then living with a man who was not her husband. To determine her character, Jesus asked her to summon her husband. When she responded truthfully by telling Jesus she had no husband, he was pleased. Jesus then displayed his omniscience by saying, "You have had five husbands."

The woman's truthfulness showed that her setback was only temporary, and Jesus was able to help her. No matter what a disciple has become, by being truthful to one's highest spiritual teacher, or guru, that disciple can be freed spiritually.

Jesus also declared himself as the Christ to the woman of Samaria. By doing so, he had one purpose: to show her that he could help her. Jesus arranged an occasion when he could see her alone because he did not want to embarrass her before his disciples. After being spiritually cleansed, the woman of Samaria became a disciple and devoted herself to the spread of Christ's teachings.

Self-honesty freed the woman of Samaria from her errors and brought her back to her rightful place as a disciple of Jesus.

Such crystal-clear self-honesty is also needed before we can face and transcend the limitations that undermine our magnetism and ability to embrace a higher destiny. In prayer or meditation, ask the Divine to show you what, if anything, is preventing you from achieving your highest goals, and then act on whatever guidance you receive. By acting with strong energy and commitment, you will strengthen your magnetism, and so be able to embrace your higher destiny.

The highest self-honesty is to strive to know our true self, to realize our innate perfection as children of God.

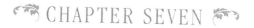

CHAPTER SEVEN

INTEGRITY

Integrity implies much more than honesty and truthfulness. It involves the full integration of every aspect of your being with your higher aspirations and beliefs.

All too often people act by following the line of least resistance, or allow their actions to be guided by social convention or others' opinions—even to the point of cutting corners ethically. Learn to heed the quiet voice of your own conscience.

Never do what others urge upon you unless your conscience endorses their advice. Seek assurance first of all in your inner self. If you fail to do so, you may someday feel you have let yourself down by accepting the priorities of others. Let your conscience tell you where your true duty lies, and don't hesitate to let it override the opinions of others. It is only to your own Higher Self that you are answerable. Always remember: intuition alone is the voice of wisdom.

Heed the quiet voice of conscience.

In February 1944, Corrie ten Boom and nearly all of her family members were arrested, betrayed by a man claiming to need their help to protect certain Jews. After being taken to the police station in Haarlem, Corrie and her family were transported by bus, along with other prisoners, to The Hague, the Gestapo's headquarters in Holland. There they were herded into a large room where, as Corrie reports, "The endless process of taking down names, addresses, and occupations began all over again." She writes that suddenly "the chief inspector's eye fell on Father."

"That old man!" he cried. "Did he have to be arrested?" . . .

"[Someone] led Father up to the desk. The Gestapo chief leaned forward. "I'd like to send you home, old fellow," he said. "I'll take your word that you won't cause any more trouble." . . .

"If I go home today," [her father answered] evenly and clearly, "tomorrow I will open my door again to any man who knocks."

Gruffly, the Gestapo chief ordered him back in line.

This was not the first time Casper ten Boom had chosen the path of integrity. After the German invasion and occupation, when the playing of the Dutch national anthem was forbidden, Casper was the first to rise to his feet when the prohibited anthem was played during a church service. The patriarch of the ten Boom clan, he opened not only his home but also his heart to anyone needing a place to hide.

Corrie would later learn that her father survived his arrest by only ten days. In his life and in his death, as we learn from Corrie's book *The Hiding Place*, Casper ten Boom *always* heeded the quiet voice of conscience.

Richard Wurmbrand: "God granted me the gift of forgetfulness."

Richard Wurmbrand (1909–2001), a man of great integrity, was a Lutheran minister in Romania when the Soviet Union took over the country in 1944. At the start of the Soviet Union's occupation of Romania, Wurmbrand began a ministry not only to his countrymen but also to Soviet soldiers. After the communist government extended its control to churches, Wurmbrand initiated an underground ministry to the Romanian people and also spoke out publicly against government control of churches. For these and other activities, he was arrested on February 29, 1948, and later imprisoned.

Richard Wurmbrand's integrity was tested countless times during his fourteen years of imprisonment. Other political prisoners were willing to inform on others in exchange for more lenient treatment: an end to discomfort, pain, or torture; better food; possible release. Subjected to cruel torture, Wurmbrand signed a statement agreeing to all the lies the communists invented about him, but nothing could persuade him to betray others. Not once did Wurmbrand even contemplate that route. He writes:

> God helped me never to say a word that harmed another. I lost consciousness easily, and they wanted me alive. . . .

> God granted me the gift of being able to forget the names of all for whom I could cause trouble. . . . I could make my mind a blank during interrogation.

Wurmbrand's integrity was founded on the bedrock of his deep faith in God. Only after being given a drug designed to weaken his will and force incriminating accusations of others, did Wurmbrand feel abandoned by Christ and begin to waver in his faith. He responded by composing a long poem celebrating his willingness to live for Christ under the harshest circumstances imaginable. Afterward, he tells us, the feeling of Christ's nearness returned, and with it, "quiet and joy."

Finally released in 1964, Wurmbrand was urged by his colleagues to leave Romania and work for religious freedom from a less dangerous location. He and his wife, Sabina, who had also been imprisoned, emigrated to America and dedicated the rest of their lives to helping Christians persecuted for their beliefs.

"I am an infidel."—The unshakeable integrity of Luther Burbank

The following statement about Luther Burbank was abridged and adapted from an article written by Paramhansa Yogananda, whose book Autobiography of a Yogi *includes a chapter on Burbank and is also dedicated to him.*

My friend Luther Burbank has passed on. I loved him dearly. He was one of the saintliest men I ever met. The keynote of his personality was love, great love. Just before his death, Burbank dramatically martyred himself by calling himself an "infidel," so that people might wake up from their sleep of superstition and seek God rationally. As Jesus offered himself for love, so Burbank was willing to be crucified by public opinion for the sake of truth. Many newspapers called Burbank an "atheist," considering him to be one more scientist without faith in God.

An atheist denies the existence of God, but an infidel is simply a disbeliever in the established religion. To a Turk, a Christian is an infidel. Yet both believe in God. The public, however, does not understand the fundamental difference between the two terms.

To most of them Burbank had denied God, but how far that is from the truth! His faith in the Great Power that rules the mighty forces of nature was the deepest chord of his being. He declared to his interviewer that he was an infidel only in the sense that Jesus was an infidel—both rebelled against prevailing systems. But let us read Burbank's actual words as recorded by the interviewer and published by the San Francisco newspaper:

Religion grows with the intelligence of man, but all religions of the past and probably all of the future will sooner or later become petrified forms .... Until that time comes, however, if religion of any name or nature makes man more happy, comfortable, and able to live peaceably with his brothers, it is good. ...

The idea that a good God would send people to a burning hell is utterly damnable to me. I don't want to have anything to do with such a God. But while I cannot conceive of such a God, I do recognize the existence of a great universal power which we cannot even begin to comprehend. ...

As for Christ—well, he has been most outrageously belied. His followers ... have so garbled his words that many of them no longer apply to present life. Christ ... was an infidel of his day because he rebelled against the prevailing religions and government. I am a lover of Christ ... and all things that help humanity ... just as he was an infidel then, I am an infidel today.

Euripides long ago said, "Who dares not speak his free thought is a slave." I nominated myself as an "infidel" as a challenge to . . . those who are asleep. The word is harmless if properly used. . .

Most of us possess discriminating reasoning powers—can we use them or must we be fed by others like babies? What does the Bible mean when it distinctly says, *By their works ye shall know them?* Works count far more than words with those who think clearly. . . .

I love everybody. I love everything. I love humanity—it has been a constant delight during all my seventy-seven years of life, and I love all the works of nature. . . . All plants, animals, and men are already in eternity traveling across the face of time. . . .

The urge toward infinite realization is in every human soul, but in some, as in Burbank, that urge is keenly felt and actively seeking fulfillment. The stupendous power that guides all creation came very close to Burbank in the course of his chosen work. He felt its overwhelming grandeur, its incomprehensible goodness and beauty.

And he knew that he, as a man, could not define or know it completely. On all subjects he kept an open mind, certain that the truth could not be so small as to be exhausted and contained in one religion, one age, or one mind.

The failure of integrity: Benedict Arnold

Benedict Arnold was an American general who betrayed his country during the Revolutionary War; his name became synonymous with the word "traitor." Arnold was born in 1741 into a respected family in Norwich, Connecticut. Although his mother came from a wealthy family, his father squandered their estate.

When the Revolutionary War broke out between Great Britain and its thirteen American colonies in 1775, Arnold joined the Continental Army. Arnold proved himself a brave and skilled leader, helping Ethan Allen's troops capture Fort Ticonderoga in 1775 and then taking part in the unsuccessful attack on British Quebec later that year, a role which earned him a promotion to brigadier general. Early in the battle to win Quebec, Arnold received a grave wound to his leg but refused to end the siege. He continued to issue orders from his sickbed.

By the latter part of 1776, Arnold had recovered sufficiently to resume his military career. He distinguished himself in campaigns at Lake Champlain, Ridgefield, and Saratoga, and gained the support of George Washington. Arnold, however, had enemies both within the military and in Congress, and despite Washington's support, political machinations and Arnold's quick temper deprived him of his due. In 1777, a group of lower-ranking men were promoted ahead of him.

During the Saratoga campaign, Arnold was wounded again in his previously injured leg. Temporarily incapable of field command, he accepted in 1778 the position of military governor of Philadelphia. That same year, Arnold married a woman of high social standing but suspected of loyalist sympathies.

Arnold and his wife led a lavish Philadelphia lifestyle, which left him with a substantial debt. Money problems and the resentment he felt over not having been promoted more quickly were factors in his fateful decision to change his allegiance and become a turncoat. He concluded that his interests would be better served assisting the British than continuing to suffer for an American army he saw as ungrateful. In May 1779, Arnold began bargaining with the British.

In 1780 Arnold was given command of West Point, the American fort on the Hudson River in New York. Arnold contacted Sir Henry Clinton, head of the British forces, and proposed handing over West Point and its men to the British. On September 21 of that year, Arnold met with British Major John Andre and made his traitorous pact, in which he was promised a large sum of money and a high position in the British Army.

However, the conspiracy was uncovered and Andre was captured and killed. Arnold fled to the enemy side and went on to lead British troops in Virginia and Connecticut.

Arnold soon became one of the most reviled figures in United States history. Ironically, his treason became, in one sense, his final service to the American cause. By 1780, Americans had grown frustrated with the slow progress toward independence and their numerous battlefield defeats. Word of Arnold's treachery helped to energize the Continental Army's sagging morale.

Arnold's treason created a negative magnetism which deprived him of the anticipated benefits of his defection to the British. Although Arnold received a commission with their army, the British never completely trusted him and he was at no time given an important military command. Arnold later moved to England, where he found no job and never received all that he had been promised by the British. He died at age sixty in London, in relative obscurity, on June 14, 1801.

"Give me liberty or give me death."

True integrity is founded on faith in God or in a transcendent principle. As the great patriot Patrick Henry declared on the eve of the American Revolution, "Give me liberty, or give me death." People of integrity are willing to sacrifice their lives rather than betray their country, their honor, or their faith in God.

Today, much of society and especially of the business world is lacking in integrity. Whatever the failings of the larger world, for us as individuals, integrity is *personal*. It must begin with *you*. How you approach your work helps define who and what you are. Loyalty to your employer is important; still more important is loyalty to honesty and truth.

When it is difficult to know what course to take, always choose a path that allows you to be a better human being. The guidelines below, followed sincerely, will assist you in determining the right course of action:

1. *Never do anything dishonest*.

Never cheat or intentionally hurt others. Your integrity is undermined by every dishonorable act. Even the willingness to indulge in a wrong act occasionally will lead, in the end, either to failure or to a complete loss of self-worth. The worst failure of all would be the loss of your own integrity.

2. *Be true to your slightest commitments*.

If you tell someone, "I will visit you next week," be sure to be there. If you say, "I will be there at eight o'clock," arrive earlier if necessary but not later. If you borrow money, make it a sacred duty to repay the debt. If you borrow a book, be sure to return it. Once you have given your word to do something, always abide by it, if only to yourself. Being true to your slightest commitments will ensure success in more serious undertakings.

3. *Never be insincere*.

Integrity means never to be insincere. A woman at a party flashed a charming smile at someone, but as soon as she turned away, her smile became a contemptuous scowl. Her obvious insincerity is the very opposite of the type of sincerity that forms the basis of integrity.

4. *Be unaffected by others' opinions.*

Integrity means to remain centered in your own understanding of what is right. A man once took his sons to a circus in Michigan. Outside, they paid the price of admission. Once inside, the management demanded that they pay again for the privilege of seats. Others meekly paid the extra price, but the father of the two boys refused this insult to his integrity. He and the two boys stood throughout the performance.

The magnetism of true integrity

Integrity involves much more than honesty and truthfulness. It means the full integration of your whole being with your higher aspirations and beliefs. Integrity includes fearlessness, kindness, inner relaxation, and cheerful acceptance of whatever comes. A person of integrity will not only be completely honest and truthful, he will be genuinely concerned for the well-being of others. He will be true, above all, to himself, in the same manner and spirit as Luther Burbank.

Let nothing tempt you to compromise an ideal. Morality is not a matter of convention. It is well-said that the Ten Commandments are engraved in human nature in tablets of light. Essential to inner peace is a clear conscience, born of facing every moral challenge from within.

CHAPTER EIGHT

SOLUTION CONSCIOUSNESS

Solution consciousness is very important for developing strong, positive magnetism. People with problem consciousness, when asked to do something, usually respond, "Yes, but ..." They assume they cannot successfully do what they are asked—that there are no solutions to their predicament. Such people rarely succeed.

We know from our earlier discussion that will power generates a flow of energy that creates a magnetic field, the basis of magnetism. Solution consciousness also is magnetic—it attracts ideas, inspirations, and other solutions from the superconscious mind. Problem consciousness, a lower level of energy, generates the type of magnetism that attracts the very problems one dreads.

This world expresses the principle of duality, of opposites: positive and negative; light and dark; pleasure and pain; joy and sorrow; success and failure. Accordingly, wherever there is a problem, there is *always* a solution. To be solution conscious means to *expect* solutions. When you are solution conscious, you develop the kind of magnetism that attracts success, and a higher force begins working in your life. More and more answers will come to you, seemingly out of the blue.

Dare to think differently.

An especially creative example of solution consciousness involved the owner of a shop whose large parking lot had become a teenage meeting place. All day long, the teenagers played on their radios loud music with a heavy beat.

The shop owner disliked the music and believed it was hurting his business, but he was not in a position to tell the youngsters to lower the volume. Instead, he came up with a positive solution: he played Mozart and other soothing classical music through a loudspeaker into the parking lot. The teenagers soon disappeared.

Solution consciousness does not mean being unaware of the problems before you. It means, rather, approaching your problems with a view toward overcoming them.

Richard Wurmbrand: "Joy can be acquired like a habit."

As discussed earlier, Richard Wurmbrand was a Christian minister who lived in communist-controlled Romania. The communists, as part of their efforts to stamp out religion, imprisoned Wurmbrand for a total of fourteen years. Wurmbrand spent three of those years in solitary confinement in a cell deep underground which allowed only three paces in each direction. A single overhead light bulb burned all night.

A man of great courage and resourcefulness, Wurmbrand found solutions that enabled him to transcend the hardships of solitary confinement. With only his thoughts for company, Wurmbrand worked out a daily routine. He slept whenever possible during the day, but stayed awake all night. And he discovered that he could spend his nights "in prayer, spiritual exercise, and praise."

He began each night with a prayer "in which tears . . . were rarely absent." Next he preached a sermon as he would in church, but in a whisper so low that no guard could hear him. It gave him courage to imagine he was surrendering his entire life to Christ; he discovered a beauty in his faith he had not previously known.

In the quiet hours he talked to his wife, Sabina, and his son, Mihai, and "pondered all that was fine and good in them." Sometimes, by concentrated thought, he sought to transmit messages to his wife, which he later learned she had received.

He learned to let go of the negative and focus only on the positive. He spent an hour each night in the mind of Colonel Dulgheru, his chief adversary and torturer, and found all sorts of excuses for him. By this means he could find it in his heart to love him. Wurmbrand entertained himself with jokes old and new. Using pieces of bread, he played chess against himself and disciplined his mind so that he would not anticipate the "other side's" next move.

At a certain point, he rarely allowed a night to pass without dancing. Dancing, he writes, "was a manifestation of joy . . . , a holy sacrifice offered before the altar of the Lord." During his three years of solitary confinement, he found that "joy can be acquired like a habit, in the same way as a folded sheet of paper falls naturally into the same fold."

"Words alone," Wurmbrand writes, "have never been able to say what man feels in the nearness of divinity. Sometimes I was so filled with joy that I felt I would burst if I did not give it expression."

There is *always* a solution.

In the depths of a hellish prison, Wurmbrand found solutions that brought joy and transcendence. Living as we do in a world of duality, of opposites, wherever a problem exists, there *must* be a solution to it. To give one example, the Native Americans learned that wherever a poisonous plant grows there is always, in its vicinity, another plant that acts as an antidote.

Direct your thoughts fearlessly toward whatever seems to you most likely to work. Know that if something you try doesn't work, something else *has* to. Such is the nature of duality. Shun the thought of failure. Always keep trying until you succeed.

George Washington Carver: "The Creator answered me."

George Washington Carver, the great African-American scientist, received his Master's Degree in Agricultural Science from Iowa State College in 1896. That same year, he accepted Booker T. Washington's invitation to take over the newly established agricultural school at Tuskegee Institute in Alabama.

When Carver wasn't teaching, he devoted himself to projects that helped Southern farmers, black and white, break the cycle of poverty and debt. Every weekend, Carver and a student loaded up a mule-drawn wagon with farm tools, seed packets, and demonstration plants, and visited black and white farmers in the backwoods and swamps. He taught them practical skills—how to raise livestock, plant vegetable gardens, preserve food, and how, through composting, to bring the depleted soil back to life. To break their economic dependence upon cotton, he encouraged them to plant peanuts.

In 1914 Carver was confronted with a major crisis. Farmers, who had heeded his advice and were producing peanuts in great abundance, suddenly discovered there was no market for their crops. Deeply upset but convinced there were solutions, Carver went to the woods in the early morning and prayed deeply for an answer. And, as he later explained, softly recounting the story, "The Creator answered me."

Back at his Tuskegee laboratory, Carver discovered over three hundred uses for the peanut, including synthetic marble, ink, glue, dye, plastics, food, oils, and milk. Within four years, Carver had helped to create a thriving market for the peanut and to transform the economy of the South.

Although few people have the genius and divine attunement to be as creatively solution conscious as Carver, all people can find, through prayer and meditation, solutions to the challenges they face. We live in a world of duality. For every problem, there is *always* a solution.

Solutions come from the superconscious mind.

There are three levels of the mind: subconscious, conscious, and superconscious. On the conscious level, we see differences. We see, for example, how people are dissimilar from trees, and how trees are distinct from rocks.

Problem consciousness arises from this sense of separateness, of concern over how to bring these separate things together in a workable way. A person with problem consciousness thinks, "How can my efforts guarantee success when that success seems to depend on other people, and on so many other things?" The answer is simple: if our will power and energy flow are strong, all of these "other things" will be drawn into that flow of energy. The conscious mind, unfortunately, does not readily grasp this principle.

The superconscious mind is solution oriented. The more we can raise our minds to a superconscious level, the more solutions will come to us—solutions we *know* are correct. All great inspirations come from superconsciousness. Meditation and prayer are the best ways to access the superconscious (see chapter 11).

Five steps toward developing solution consciousness

1. *Learn to say "yes" to life.*

There is in everyone a "no-saying" tendency as well as a "yes-saying" inclination. The "no-saying" tendency draws the mind down into the realm of negativity and judgment. Only when you have overcome the negative, critical spirit can you uplift your mind into the attunement needed to receive answers from the superconscious.

2. *Be convinced a solution exists.*

Every problem has a solution. Hold onto that conviction. Don't dwell on difficulties longer than it takes to define them clearly. Any doubt arising from subconscious habits will act as static and prevent a clear flow from superconsciousness.

3. *Always be practical.*

Although it's important to be practical, you should never equate practicality with negativity. To see things clearly is to be realistic, not negative. You become negative when you have a wish or a feeling against something. A person with solution consciousness, while certainly aware of possible problems, instead of dwelling on what could go wrong, thinks, "What can I do to make things turn out *right?*"

4. *Lovingly demand an answer.*

Focus your mind at the point between the eyebrows and form in your mind a clear idea of the kind of solution you want. Lovingly demand an answer to your question. Make the demand with solution consciousness, in full expectation of receiving an immediate answer.

Attracting higher guidance does not depend on the time spent seeking it. What is important is *focused* energy. Focused energy generates the magnetism to attract whatever guidance it seeks.

5. *"God helps those who help themselves."*

The way to draw higher assistance is to put yourself in attunement with the Divine through prayer and meditation. If your will power is strong and your energy positive, focused, and practical, a Higher Power will often step in and help you. Because you have done your best, the Divine will enter the picture. (This subject is explored further in chapter 11.)

There *has* to be a solution.

Try to mix with people who find solutions to their challenges and succeed in their efforts. Make it a point to keep at a distance people who obsess with problems. Otherwise, you risk being pulled down by the lower energy of their problem consciousness, an attitude which often degenerates into failure consciousness.

The people who find answers in life are not the so-called hard-headed realists who are always thinking of what is wrong and why nothing will work. Those who find answers are *always* the ones who are absolutely convinced that there *has* to be a solution, that *something* can be done.

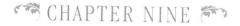

CHAPTER NINE

NONATTACHMENT

One of the basic teachings in the Bhagavad Gita is *nish-kam karma*: action without desire for the fruits of action—nonattachment. People who concentrate on the fruits of their actions often go from one desire to another; they frequently become enmeshed in earthly desires. At the same time, everyone needs enough material prosperity, health, and opportunity not to fall victim to excessive material concerns. In other words, even if our main goals in life are spiritual, we must be able to fulfill our material needs. The question is: How best to do both?

Books that teach how to actualize our ideas often stress the importance of visualizing clearly the exact description of the thing we want. Do we want a car? Then visualize the model and color of car we wish for, perhaps even seeing ourselves sitting in it with the keys in the ignition. Some of these books also encourage us to desire *intensely* whatever we want, arguing that intensity of feeling will help draw the object of our desire.

Keep in mind, however, that when desire and attachment exist, what we attract may not be what we need, or may be much less than could have come to us. Indeed, an exclusive focus on one possibility could easily blind us to other more desirable options. The following story illustrates the blinding effects of desire and attachment.

The heavenly junkyard: rejected gifts

A man had just died and St. Peter was showing him around paradise. They came to what St. Peter called the "heavenly junk yard."

"Here you'll find all the gifts from heaven," he explained, "that people on earth rejected."

"Why, that's impossible!" exclaimed the newcomer. "Some of these things are beautiful. Look at that Cadillac over there. Who could possibly have rejected that?"

"Well, it's interesting that you should ask about that particular car," replied St. Peter. "As it happens, you were the one who rejected that Cadillac."

"Impossible!" protested the man. "I'd never have refused such a wonderful gift."

"All the same, it was you," St. Peter replied. "You see, the Cadillac was ready and waiting to be delivered to you, but every time you prayed for a car, you kept visualizing a Volkswagen."

Focus on the energy flow, not the objective.

It is important to keep in mind that magnetism is a flow of energy—and that energy flows much more forcefully when we think of it as fluid, without fixed and definite goals. When putting out effort to achieve a goal, it is much better to focus on the *energy flow* itself, not the specific objective, even when our need is for a specific sum of money. Although it is possible to attract a specific goal by focusing on it intensely, what we attract may end up being not only *less* than we could have had, but something we do not truly need.

Swami Kriyananda offers an instructive example of how to achieve a goal by focusing on the energy flow. In the early years of Ananda Village, during the 1970s, members were pledging different amounts of money to improve certain areas of the community. Even though he did not have the money at the time, Kriyananda secretly pledged $2500 to pave the entrance to the village—the largest project on the list. The money was needed in two weeks.

When Kriyananda later prayed about the request, he mentioned the specific sum of money needed, but he did not *visualize* any sum or *how* the money might come. Instead, he concentrated on the *strength of the energy* he was focusing on the prayer and the purpose the money was to serve (paving the entrance). Then, with great will power, he projected that strong flow of energy upward from his heart and out through his spiritual eye.

One morning, nearly two weeks later, he found an envelope on the floor near his front door. In it was a letter from a friend who had formerly lived at Ananda and who had recently received an inheritance. The envelope also contained a check for three thousand dollars. Kriyananda writes that "when you act with nonattachment, you can be sure of one thing: when success comes, it will be in the best possible way."

How to formulate a prayer demand

The approach used by Swami Kriyananda breaks down into the following five steps:

1. When praying about your request, mention very clear-

ly what it is you need.

2. Focus the energy of your request at your heart and also at the spiritual eye, the point between the eyebrows.

3. Calling on the universe to reinforce your energy, send a strong flow of energy up from the heart and out through the point between the eyebrows. Invest your request with all of your energy.

4. Concentrate more on the strength and magnetic power of your outflowing energy than on the particular object or situation you hope to influence by your demand.

5. Make God your partner in this undertaking, and offer up the fruits of your efforts to Him, seeking to please Him alone.

A warning against selfish motive

Nishkam karma, acting without desire for the fruits of action, is not a prohibition against action. It is a warning against acting with selfish motive. Acting with nonattachment does not mean neglecting our families or other material duties, but performing those duties with the desire to please God or to serve others, or both. Selfishness of any type separates us from the divine reality that sustains all life; it ultimately limits our ability to attract success.

With an attitude of nonattachment we are able to respond to life according to what is right rather than what pleases us. Whether we succeed is in God's hands, not ours. Approaching life with this attitude imparts a great deal more freedom than thinking, "I *have* to make it work." Our job is simply to keep trying, and to do our best.

To work with nonattachment is to live more in the moment. It is to define ourselves by the effort, not the result.

Usually in front of us is a specific task which, when completed, will be followed by another task. An attitude of nonattachment frees us from scattering our energy in emotional ups and downs and allows us to ask, "What am I supposed to do in *this very moment?*" Nonattachment brings peace and contentment. Attachments, on the other hand, cause one to live in fear, remorseful about the past and worried about the future.

The more nonattached we are, the freer we are to enjoy the present. It was these qualities of nonattachment and contentment that Joseph Cornell, a well-known naturalist, displayed when he found himself lost in the Sierra Nevadas.

Lost in the wilderness: nonattached and inwardly free

"It was late spring, and snow still covered the Sierra Nevada high country. While hiking back to my car, I went down the wrong side of a ridge and into unfamiliar territory.

"There wasn't enough daylight left to retrace my steps. Because I didn't have a coat it was imperative that I get to lower elevation and warmer, snow-free ground. I knew that continuing my present course would eventually bring me to a road—if not that night, certainly by morning.

"Though I realized that I might have some challenges ahead, I felt completely relaxed. I focused my mind on God and offered myself into His hands. Knowing that fear and imagination often cause unwise decisions, I was determined to remain calm and centered in the presence of God. As I did so, I found my walk becoming more and more joyful.

"Well after sundown I reached a large lake and began walking along its shore. When it was almost dark, I saw in the distance two men fishing from a boat. I wanted to ask them where I was but because yelling such a long way would disturb my inner peace, I kept on walking, feeling God's presence, which was the only thing that seemed important.

"When I came to a small cove, I saw another fisherman on the far bank. Now I was able to ask him in a calm, normal voice the name of the lake. 'Spaulding,' he replied. I was familiar with this lake; I now knew where I was.

"Minutes later, one of the fishermen asked, 'Why don't you know the name of the lake?' When I calmly explained how I had come to the lake by mistake, the man exclaimed, 'But your car is twelve miles away, and it's nighttime! We'll drive you there.'

"My fisherman's friends disagreed with this plan. I was feeling so free and blissful inside that I didn't want the night to end. I sat in the backseat of their car, comfortably letting things unfold, as they discussed quite energetically whether to drive me or not. I felt perfectly fine with whatever they decided.

"My friend and advocate eventually convinced his friends to drive me to my car. While driving my own car home that night, I felt deeply grateful to God for helping me experience the joy of accepting life's circumstances and not allowing time-consciousness to destroy my serenity."[*]

Nonattachment and solution consciousness

The question arises: What is the relationship between nonattachment and solution-consciousness? The more attached we are to a situation in need of changing, the more

---

[*] Adapted from *AUM: The Melody of Love*, Crystal Clarity Publishers. (Joseph Cornell is the author of a number of books, including *Sharing Nature: Nature Activities for All Ages*.)

difficult it will be for us to identify the solution that will change that situation in the best possible way. If, for example, a financial depression comes and the best solution to our decreased income is to sell the house of our dreams, we must be nonattached enough 1) to understand that selling the house is, in fact, the best solution, and 2) to go forward and sell the house.

For Joseph Cornell, who was lost in the wilderness, nonattachment was a way of life, based on his faith in God. His solution was to do what he could to help himself and then to offer his life into God's hands, in the firm conviction that, by so doing, he would be protected.

Try to practice nonattachment on a daily basis. When an experience comes that you do not like, try to accept it calmly and appreciate its hidden lesson. Simply say, "Thank you, God. I give any sense of attachment back to You." The fruit of nonattachment is ever-increasing inner freedom. And always remember: energy used joyfully and willingly generates *more* energy.

Five steps to greater nonattachment

1. *Balance nonattachment with compassion*. Some yoga practitioners embrace the negative aspects of nonattachment and hold themselves aloof from other people and their concerns. When nonattachment is limited to a rejecting frame of mind, it can easily develop into spiritual pride. It is therefore important to balance nonattachment with compassion.

2. *Increase your attachment to God*. Nature abhors a

vacuum. Instead of negatively trying to remove attachments, substitute for them a better attachment—to God's love and joy.

3. *Develop a giving frame of mind*. True nonattachment requires an expansion of identity, a sense of kinship with others. A step toward that goal is to meditate, harmonize the vibrations in your heart, and then radiate only positive vibrations outward to the world around you. This practice puts you in a giving frame of mind. The more you give and the less you desire for yourself, the more you will find yourself sustained by life itself.

4. *Avoid poverty consciousness.* If possible, show your appreciation to those who improve the quality of life by the way they live and dress. Doing so puts you in an expansive frame of mind, which will help offset the contractive energy of poverty consciousness.

5. *Live in this world as a guest*. Always remember that this world is not your home. You are here temporarily, as the great yogi Lahiri Mahasaya put it, as a guest. By trying generously to improve the quality of life on earth, you will also uplift yourself.

The following two practices will help you develop nonattachment and even-mindedness.

An inner fire ceremony: Before going to bed at night, visualize a fire at the point between the eyebrows and offer into the flames everything in your life: possessions, emotions, likes and dislikes, your very life. Offer all those things you are reluctant to give up: money, relationships, job, health, your children. For most people these are usually the strongest attachments. You can also practice this visualization as you wake up, especially if you are anxious or worried.

The heart as a golden ball: Visualize your heart as a golden ball with strings protruding from it, each string representing an attachment. Cut away the strings, no matter how thick, until the golden ball is completely free of strings. Then polish the ball until it is bright and shiny. Doing this visualization two or three times a day will not only help you develop nonattachment, it will also cleanse your aura and strengthen your devotion.

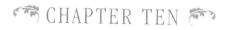

CHAPTER TEN

THE LAW OF KARMA

Karma is supreme, far more than most people realize. Every human tendency is the result of an individual choice, exercised either in this life or in former lives. People are moved forward on the path to enlightenment by the law of karma. Every action, every thought, reaps its corresponding reward. If people fail to act in harmony with their higher nature, they experience pain and suffering. They have attracted that suffering by the magnetism projected by their karma. If, on the other hand, they act in harmony with their higher nature, they will experience increasing inner peace and happiness.

Most people are controlled by their habits. Although they themselves created those habits through deeds performed in the past, a habit, once formed, is self-perpetuating. People seldom think of their habitual actions as bad. Whatever they do seems, at least to them, well-intentioned. But if their actions create disharmony for others, those waves will inevitably return as disharmony directed at *them*.

Deflecting negative karma: "A superhuman effort of will"

Success depends not only upon our will power and energy in this lifetime but also upon our past-life successes and failures, which have been carried over into the present as subconscious karmic tendencies. Successful people may sometimes experience reverses in their fortunes because of the sudden manifestation of subconscious failure tendencies. Such was the experience of Henry Ford.

Paramhansa Yogananda explained that Henry Ford nearly lost his business and entire fortune during World War I because of failure tendencies from past lives. Ford had undoubtedly been prosperous in former lives, and he had acquired great wealth, but his subconscious mind was filled with failure tendencies owing to losses in other lives. During the war, when conditions were unfavorable to certain lines of business, his failure seeds sprouted and nearly caused his financial ruin. If he had allowed himself to become discouraged, he would have lost everything.

By a superhuman effort of will, Ford was able to fight off brutal business competitors who were determined to destroy the organization he had built during years of hard work. His success consciousness from the past—reinforced by his positive attitude, perseverance, initiative, trained business judgment, and skill in choosing the right workers—enabled him to prevail.

Accept responsibility for your karma.

Faced with the prospect of losing his business, Henry Ford took full responsibility for the reversal in his fortunes and devoted his full will power and energy to saving his business. Unfortunately, many people, faced with a similar need to accept responsibility for their karma, seek refuge in the thought that they are innocent victims of an implacable fate.

The root causes of our karma grow out of sight in the subconscious mind. We ourselves have put down those roots by wrong deeds performed in the past. If anyone behaves wrongly toward us, it is because we have *attracted* that behavior by our past actions. The magnetism of our karma has drawn that hurtful behavior to us. If misfortune befalls us, we must try not to blame anyone. The way to transcend negative karma is 1) to accept responsibility for whatever misfortunes we encounter, 2) to devote our full will power and energy to changing the situation, and 3) to do our best to eliminate whatever attitudes or tendencies in our nature attracted that karma to us.

Karma can always be mitigated. If, for example, our karma is darkened by dishonesty, we can improve it by being rigidly honest from now on. Frank W. Abagnale's life offers an especially instructive example of how such a change can be accomplished.

Mitigating karma: The example of Frank Abagnale

Frank W. Abagnale, whose story is told in the book and subsequent movie *Catch Me If You Can*, was a millionaire twice over before he was twenty-one. His wealth was based entirely on stolen money—money which he used to support a luxurious lifestyle.

Growing up, Abagnale lived in an upper-middle-class home in Bronxville, New York. His parents divorced when he was fourteen, and Abagnale chose to live with his father, a successful businessman and politician who spent a fair amount of time in New York's finest saloons. Although he did not drink, young Abagnale often joined his father in the taverns. Abagnale's early delinquencies, one of which involved the misuse of his father's credit card, landed him in a school for problem boys in the Bronx, but to little avail. After a bad-check-writing spree, Abagnale left home at age sixteen. Over six feet tall, broad shouldered, and weighing 170 pounds, he looked considerably older.

Frank Abagnale went on to become one of the most daring con men in history. His brief criminal career included masquerading as an airline pilot, as the supervising resident of a hospital, as an attorney at law, and as a college sociology professor. At age twenty-one, after cashing more than two and a half million dollars in forged checks, he was captured and sent to prison.

Abagnale writes that he "had reached the pinnacle of a criminal mountain and the view wasn't . . . great." Even before he was caught, he yearned for a quiet life. Just when he thought he had found such a life in a small town in France, an airline stewardess recognized him and alerted the police. He was imprisoned for six years, including six months in a French prison where he was subjected to inhuman, life-threatening conditions.

After paying his debt to society, Abagnale decided to direct his expertise in "the mechanics of forgery, check swindling, counterfeiting, and similar crimes . . . into the right channels." Perhaps unknowingly, Abagnale began to mitigate his bad karma by using his knowledge to help banks and financial institutions protect themselves against the kinds of crimes he himself had committed.

Today Abagnale is one of the world's most respected authorities on counterfeiting and secure documents. For twenty-five years, he worked with the FBI Financial Crimes Unit. He teaches, at the FBI's National Academy, a program that instructs local, state, and federal law enforcement agencies nationwide. The founder of a secure documents corporation based in Washington D.C., Abagnale lectures regularly throughout the world.

Frank Abagnale's life is an example of how we can mitigate a karmic debt by putting out a strong *opposing* energy. We can mitigate the karma of unkindness and negativity, for example, by making a conscious effort to be kind to others generally or by sending thoughts of love and kindness to specific people. We can mitigate the karma of dishonesty by becoming scrupulously honest in all business dealings and by making truthfulness a priority in all areas of life, both personal and professional.

Frank Abagnale was an immature sixteen-year-old when he embarked on his life of crime. Surely his thirty-year effort to help prevent the kinds of crimes he himself had committed has balanced at least some of the bad karma accrued during his brief life of crime.

Indomitable will power: The man who found gold twice

We don't have to be a slave to bad karma. It was energy we ourselves put out in the past that created that karma, but if we change directions now and, with a great deal of energy, express a strong positive magnetism, we can offset the negative results of that energy. The following true story illustrates how a strong, focused will power, combined with a positive attitude, can defeat even the harshest karma.

A certain gold prospector in America lived with his wife in a humble cabin in the mountains. For years he found only enough gold to make ends meet. Undaunted, he kept on prospecting, hoping someday to strike it rich. Throughout that time, he and his wife kept a positive, cheerful outlook on life.

Finally the man did strike gold and, that same day, sold his claim to a mining company. He arrived home with a large bag of money; he and his wife were now *very* rich. The prospector gave the money to his wife and later, with her consent, went out to celebrate with a few of his friends. Meanwhile his wife hid the money in the wood stove, which they rarely used because of their limited resources.

When her husband arrived home with his friends, he invited them in. It was late, and the air was chilly. He placed a few logs in the stove as quietly as possible, and built a fire. The blaze consumed their fortune in cash. The next morning, upon discovering that all of their newly acquired wealth had gone up in flames, the woman was devastated. Her husband, fortunately, remained calm and positive. That very same day he struck another vein of gold, much richer than the first.

The key point of this story is the importance of meeting adversity with indomitable will power and a positive attitude. If you never allow adversity, no matter how appalling, to weaken your will power or to cause you to become discouraged, your positive magnetism will enable you to transcend even the harshest karma. Always remember: "like attracts like." The more positive energy you put out, the more positive energy you will attract.

Mass karma and individual karma: "You've got to come see us now."

There is a difference between individual and mass karma, sometimes referred to as group karma. When an airplane crashes and everyone on the airplane is killed, mass karma is involved, but it does not necessarily mean that everyone on the plane also had the *individual* karma to die. A person would be drawn into that mass karma only if he or she did not have a strong enough *individual* karma to offset the group karma and live.

As an example, before the atomic bomb fell on Hiroshima, many residents of that city received urgent letters from relatives saying, "You've got to come see us *now.*" Those Hiroshima residents were removed from the scene because it was not their karma to die, and also because their individual karma to live was strong enough to protect them from that mass karma. A person *without* a strong enough individual karma to live would have been drawn into the group karma.

People living in a particular country usually have to bear the karma of that country even though it may not be their individual karma. However, like those removed from the scene at Hiroshima, if they are strong spiritually, they will not have to bear that country's karma. Their strong spiritual magnetism will protect them from that mass karma by preventing any darkness from penetrating their auras.

Freedom from the dictates of karma

Although the law of karma functions to a great extent automatically, it is also guided by a universal intelligence and love, and can be intelligently diverted. Hence, the concept of divine grace. Grace can be won above all by love for God and devotion to Him. The more we give generously of ourselves to God and to life, the more karmic law supports us in return. Those who seek prosperity only for themselves are destined to be poor for some time; those who think of others and work for group prosperity will be supported and guided by cosmic forces in their efforts to achieve success.

Seek to be guided from within, attuned to the Divine, the infinite power and wisdom behind karmic law. The more you live from within, and the less your actions are motivated by egoic desires, the greater will be your control over the outer events in your life. Through meditation and your unfolding awareness of yourself as a soul, you will begin to free yourself from the dictates of all karma. With the attainment of Self-realization (oneness with the Divine), which is the ultimate destiny of every soul, you will be released forever from the bondage of karmic law.

The following story by Paramhansa Yogananda provides an excellent overview of the law of karma, and illustrates the karmic consequences of good and bad actions. It also answers these common questions about how the law works:

1. Is karma always fair?
2. Why do good people have bad karma?
3. Why do things go well for villainous people?
4. Can karma be changed?
5. How can we offset bad karma?

Why the Rich Man Became Poor and the Poor Man Became Rich

There once lived in India two friends—Mr. Sham, a rich man, and Mr. Honest, a poor man. Both lived with their families in a large double house. Mr. Sham was a shameless rogue and a dissolute individual, whereas Mr. Honest was a very upright, religious man. Their modes of living could in no way explain their different destinies in life.

Mr. Sham was unfaithful to his wife and indulged in unbridled sin, yet he had a loyal, beautiful, spiritual wife who put up with his cruel ways. It seemed that the more Mr. Sham sinned and caroused, the more he prospered and grew strong and healthy. On the other hand, Mr. Honest was strictly loyal to his wife, even though she was homely, nagging, and unfaithful. Yet, it seemed that the more Mr. Honest absorbed himself in metaphysics and meditation, the worse his misfortunes became. Loss of friends, bad investments, and extreme poverty doggedly pursued him.

Mr. Sham often said, "Look here, Mr. Honest. If you will forsake this religious and metaphysical nuttiness, I will give you a financial start and you will then attract riches and friends."

"I can show you that God exists and responds to prayers."

In reply Mr. Honest would remonstrate, saying, "Nay, my friend. Thank you for your offer, but I have no intention of giving up my virtuous ways, which give me an inner satisfaction even though they do not yield a harvest of wealth and prosperity."

One evening Mr. Sham forced the issue with Mr. Honest in the house parlor. He gravely said, "Don't you see that I live a natural life? I take a drink when I want it. I do what my impulses move me to do—and see, I am as healthy and happy as a lark. Your metaphysics have paralyzed your will power and creative ability, and have mixed you up. Your sick mind keeps you physically and financially ill. Give up God and follow me, and you will be happy. There is no God, and there are no laws of life except what you create."

Mr. Honest, beside himself with wrath, shouted, "You ignorant man, there is a God and He listens to prayers! He has mysterious ways of rewarding His devotees after they pass His earthly tests. I would wager that I can show you God exists and that He responds to prayers."

Mr. Sham shot back a quick challenge. "Well, Mr. Super-Favorite of a Nonexistent God, why don't you coax your Almighty Nothingness with your prayers to demonstrate something tangible to me?"

With perfect assurance, Mr. Honest answered, "All right, I accept your challenge. I will start praying to God night and day for a month. I am confident He will answer my prayer through all that happens to you and me on Friday, a month from now."

Mr. Sham retorted, "What do you mean by 'all that happens to you and me on Friday a month from now'?"

Mr. Honest responded, "If God sends fortune to you and misfortune to me on that Friday, then you win and we shall know there is no God. But if He sends fortune to me and misfortune to you, then you will know that God exists and has responded to my prayers. If I lose, I will follow your ways of living, and if you lose, you must follow mine."

Mr. Sham burst into a torrent of laughter and said, "All right, Archangel, I will wait for your prayers to bring God's action on the appointed Friday. And remember, if I win, you must follow my natural ways of living."

"Heavenly Father, please punish Sham and bring me good fortune."

Mr. Honest prayed night and day for a month in the following manner: "Heavenly Father, my own dear God, if You exist, please punish Sham on that Friday and bring me good fortune, so that I may win for Your sake."

When the telltale Friday arrived, Mr. Sham was in high spirits. He felt he was sure to win the bet and, led by a strange hunch, went to a nearby forest to hunt. Ruthlessly, he killed more birds than he needed to feed his family and packed them on his horse. On his way home, Mr. Sham stopped under a shady tree to rest. As he lay on the ground, he began to strike absentmindedly at the sod with his knife. Suddenly he heard a metallic sound. Curious, he began to dig and struck an iron chest. Opening the lid, to his amazement he beheld three million dollars in pirate-plundered gold coins.

Mr. Sham was beside himself with joy and, emptying his sacks of the dead birds, filled them with the gold coins. On his arrival home, to his great astonishment and merriment, he heard that Mr. Honest, while walking in a prayerful mood, had nearly been killed through a collision with a horse and carriage, and had been carried unconscious to the hospital.

Exultingly Mr. Sham said to himself, "Now I know that there is no God. I hope Mr. Honest recovers from his accident and lives long enough to realize this."

On his return from the hospital, Mr. Honest heard about his friend's luck. In response, that same Friday afternoon, he threw all his metaphysical books into the fire and rushed out of the house into the forest, determined to end his life. He could not believe in God any longer, but neither could he relinquish virtue or deliberately become evil. So he went to a lake in the jungle and was tying himself to a heavy stone to drown himself when God sent a plainly dressed saint to explain matters.

"Mr. Honest, you could not bribe God with your prayers."

The saint gently but firmly accosted him, "Mr. Honest, what are you doing here on this glorious God-ordained day?"

Mr. Honest angrily replied, "Get away. It is none of your business what I am doing. I don't ever again want to hear that meaningless word, 'God,' again."

To this the saint responded, "Why? Is it because you bet about God and lost by being run over by a horse and carriage?" Mr. Honest was astonished that this stranger knew all of these facts.

Softening, he said, "Honored sir, can you tell me why I, who have zealously studied metaphysics and faithfully meditated, should grow physically and financially poorer in every way. Why did God not only turn a deaf ear to my prayer, but make a fool of me before Mr. Sham, seemingly proving to him the truth of atheism?"

The saint replied, "Mr. Honest, you could not bribe God by your prayers. You must never bet about God, and whenever you pray, you must not decide that He has to answer your prayers. You should depend upon His wisdom to determine whether your prayers should be fulfilled.

"In your past incarnation you were a great sinner, and thus sick all the time. You made up your mind to be a virtuous man only just before your death. That is why in this life you were born with a strong resolution to study metaphysics and to meditate. But because you were a sinner before, you have met with many physical, mental, and spiritual reverses in this life. In your previous life, you also had a very good, forgiving wife whom you never appreciated, and tortured with your evil ways.

"For all the sins of your past life it was ordained that on Friday you were to die, but because you have been virtuous in this life, your life was spared and you escaped with only an accident. All the evil seeds of your past actions have now sprouted and are dead, and the balance of virtue in you has become greater than that of evil. Return home, and henceforth luck will seek you in everything."

"Forgive my ignorant blasphemies against You."

Mr. Honest sobbed with gratitude and, looking up to heaven, burst forth, "Oh God, my Beloved, I crave your pardon. Forgive my ignorant blasphemies against You."

Then Mr. Honest inquired, "Honored saint, will you satisfy my curiosity as to why all good things were attracted to Mr. Sham, and why even on that particular Friday he found three million dollars?"

"Well, my son," the saint replied, "Mr. Sham in his past life was a tolerably virtuous man, but in time became tired of his virtuous life and made up his mind to live according to his evil impulses. And it was just about then that he died. So, Mr. Sham was born a sinner due to his resolution before death. But because he was virtuous for most of his last incarnation, he automatically reaped the results of his past good actions. Thus he attracted to himself a good wife, friends, fortune, and health.

"Now, however, the balance is turned and the sins of this life have grown heavier than his past virtue. The treasure he received that Friday is nothing compared to the imperishable virtue you have acquired in this life by constant hard labor."

Saying this, the saint vanished. Mr. Honest returned home

to find his nagging wife stricken with a terrible disease. After she died, he met a sweet and spiritual woman, whom he married. His ill health disappeared and he received a large inheritance from a rich aunt, who had changed her will a few hours before her death.

On the other hand, Mr. Sham found himself suddenly stricken with paralysis. Shortly after this, his wife died. Mr. Sham had buried all of his money in a secret chamber beneath the floor under his bed, but a disgruntled servant got scent of it and arranged for masked robbers to steal the money while Mr. Sham lay helpless. After that, Mr. Sham lived the rest of his life on the charity of his friend, Mr. Honest.

Lessons from the foregoing story:

1. Both good and bad karma often intensify on the eve of a shift in karmic fortunes. This principle explains why, shortly before their karma changed, Mr. Sham found buried treasure and Mr. Honest was nearly killed in a collision.

2. In turning to God, we should pray with nonattachment and not presume that He must answer our prayers in the way we decide.

3. Bad karma can be greatly mitigated by devotion to God and by virtuous living.

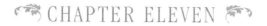

CHAPTER ELEVEN

ATTUNEMENT WITH THE
INFINITE CONSCIOUSNESS

The possibility of success is greatly increased through attunement with the Infinite Consciousness, the vast intelligence that underlies all life, what we usually refer to as God or the Divine. To act in *conscious* attunement with that Infinite Consciousness means to recognize that we are already part of that vast reality, and that by acting in attunement with it, we can achieve far more in life than by relying on our own limited powers.

In earlier chapters of this book, we have given a number of examples of the intervention of the Divine in human affairs, including instances when that assistance came uninvited. These examples are powerful testimony to the truth that the Infinite Consciousness is *just that*: infinitely conscious in every atom of creation, in every situation imaginable, and in every aspect of a limitless reality beyond our human ability to comprehend.

"I will just keep trying."

A dramatic example of divine intervention without conscious invitation involves a mountain climber who had grown up in Yugoslavia and had made many first ascensions by climbing to the top of mountains no one else had scaled. He was thus highly skilled as a mountain climber when he decided to climb a mountain from an approach never before attempted. Although most sides of this mountain were relatively easy to ascend, this one was so difficult that no one had ever attempted it.

He was almost to the top of the mountain when he discovered something he hadn't been able to see from below: the mountain bulged outward. The only way to get beyond the outward bulge was to climb upside down for a few moments, a physically impossible feat. It was also impossible for him to descend the mountain from his present position.

Logically, the man had no choice but to sit there until he died. Calmly he thought, "Rather than starving to death, I will just keep trying." Every time he climbed beyond the bulge, he fell back onto the ledge. After each failed attempt he thought, "I might as well die of bruises as of hunger," and kept going. After twenty-five or thirty attempts, as he again tried to climb past the bulge, he felt a force suddenly push him against the mountain and hold him there until he reached the top. From there he could easily climb down the other side.

Important aspects of magnetism are involved in that mountain climber's success: strong will power, focused energy, a positive attitude, solution consciousness, and nonattachment. Though death loomed as a distinct possibility, he did not panic and give up. With inner calmness he chose the strategy that ultimately saved his life. This extraordinary story also shows that when we do our very best, we generate the magnetism to attract divine assistance. Although that assistance sometimes comes uninvited, and in ways that can only be described as "miraculous," the main means of invoking the support and guidance of the Divine are meditation and prayer.

Attuning to the Infinite Consciousness: meditation

Meditation is the most direct route to attuning to the Infinite Consciousness. It is also the most direct path to every type of success, spiritual or material. Regular meditation calms the mind, making it receptive to inspiration from the Infinite Consciousness.

Some of Paramhansa Yogananda's most highly advanced disciples were successful businessmen. They brought strong powers of concentration to their efforts to achieve business success, and later applied that same intensity of focus to meditation and their spiritual search. Rajarshi Janakananda (James J. Lynn), Paramhansa Yogananda's most highly advanced disciple and his spiritual successor, was a successful businessman with many responsibilities, and also chairman of several boards of directors. Even so, he devoted his morning hours to meditation. A frequent visitor to Yogananda's retreat in Southern California, he would spend hours seated on the lawn in deep meditation.

The more we attune ourselves to the Infinite Consciousness through meditation, the more effective we become in every area of life. Whenever you need guidance or understanding, meditate and go within. When your mind is calm, ask the Divine to direct you to the right course of action, and then act on the guidance you receiveT. Start first by seeking guidance on less significant matters, gradually working up to more important issues. A gradual approach will protect you from the mistake of believing you have received guidance on matters of great importance, only to find out later it was your imagination or personal desire. Although meditation requires commitment and effort, even a little practice brings a sense of confidence and well-being.

For many people, one of the main obstacles to effective meditation is restlessness, the inability to rid the mind of distracting thoughts and impressions. Indeed, if your mind is not practiced at concentration, the mere resolution *not* to think of something may cause you to think of nothing but that something, as illustrated by the following story.

"Be sure not to think about monkeys."

There was a spiritual seeker who went to a saint and asked to be taught to meditate. "I want to achieve cosmic consciousness and find God immediately!" the young man declared. "How hard will I have to work at it?"

"Oh, you won't have to work at all," the saint assured him with a smile. He meant (though he didn't say so), that "work" wasn't the right word, since it implies tension; "conscious relaxation" fits the case better. Therefore he added: "Simply sit erect on a straight chair in a darkened room, facing east with your eyes closed. Banish all thoughts from your mind and focus your attention at the point between the eyebrows while chanting 'AUM.'"

The new student was delighted; so little work, for such vast results! Just as he was about to leave the room, the saint called to him, "Oh, by the way, there's something I forgot to add. While engaged in this practice, be sure not to think about monkeys."

"That's easy," the student replied. "I never think of monkeys."

A week later the young man returned. "Take back your technique, Master," he exclaimed. "Tell me," the saint replied with a smile. "What happened?"

"When I got home and sat to meditate, the first thing that came into my mind was, 'I must not think about monkeys!' I then proceeded to consider every kind of monkey that can be found in India.

"By the second night I'd exhausted all the Indian monkeys, so I went to an encyclopedia and researched the different kinds of monkeys in Africa, South America, Indonesia, Malaya, and Northern Australia. I've become an expert on monkeys, but meditation has not given me a moment's peace! The only thing it has given me is 'monkey consciousness!' Therefore I say: take back your technique."

The saint laughed heartily. "You see? I was trying to show you how untrained your concentration is. Until you can make your mind obey you, you cannot achieve *any* form of success, not to mention success in the art of meditation.

"Deep meditation isn't *work*, as such, though it does require deep effort. What you need to do is relax your mind from restless thoughts. Just *relax*, absorbing yourself deeply in what you are doing. When concentrating at the point between the eyebrows, try to focus positively on one thing at a time, with full attention. And don't try *not* to think of anything!"

Meditation strengthens our magnetism.

Success in meditation depends not only on our current efforts but also on our karma, which can impede positive results. The solution is to continue trying, knowing that sincere, ongoing efforts will inevitably bring success. Indeed, the conscientious practice of meditation strengthens qualities and practices that, in themselves, are essential aspects of magnetism, and that ultimately will bring success not only in meditation but in all areas of life:

Will Power: Daily meditation greatly strengthens our will power, giving us the strength of will necessary to succeed in whatever we undertake.

Concentration: Meditation strengthens our concentration, enabling us to resolve issues more quickly, without the need for extended reflection.

Enthusiasm: Enthusiasm may be defined as the spirit of joy channeled through the power of the will. The more we experience God's joy in meditation, the more perfectly does our enthusiasm express His joy.

Kindness: Kindness toward others unfolds naturally as we try through meditation to attune to and live by the highest in us.

Positive Attitudes: Meditation is the best way to harmonize our emotions. Increasingly, no matter how people respond to us, we will be able to maintain our inner peace.

Honesty: Meditation strengthens our capacity to accept what is and not to wish things to be other than they are.

Truthfulness: Through meditation we learn to speak only the *beneficial* truth where others are concerned and also to see where we ourselves need to change.

Integrity: Meditation gives us the moral vigor to stand by truth whatever the cost to us personally.

Solution Consciousness: Meditation makes us more solution oriented. We approach our problems with perfect confidence that a solution exists.

Nonattachment: Meditation enables us to relinquish attachments to human fulfillments in the deepening understanding that nothing is really ours, and that our true home is in God.

The importance of devotion

The example of the saints shows that the most powerful magnetism comes from attunement with the Divine, including the magnetism to work miracles. Essential to that attunement is devotion. To meditate and pray deeply, devotion is essential.

Devotion is love for God. Since God *is* love and like attracts like, devotion to God put us on the divine wavelength and enables us to draw the divine consciousness into ourselves.

Heartfelt chanting is one of the best ways to open the heart in devotion. To draw a divine response, an experience of the Divine's inner presence, the chanting must be quiet and inward, not boisterous or loud.

Mental whispers: A quiet inward feeling

During a play based on the life of Krishna, the well-known avatar of ancient India, the audience could see two open rooms with a divider between them. Krishna was alone in one of the rooms. In the other room some of his followers were loudly singing and dancing to the accompaniment of drums and cymbals, hoping to attract Krishna's attention. Failing to do so, they stopped playing after a while and left the room. Radha, one of Krishna's closest disciples, then entered the room, sat down, and in a near-whisper said,

"Oh, Krishna." Because she had called to him with devotion, Krishna at once stopped what he was doing and ran to be with Radha.

True devotion is a deep, quiet, inward feeling, not something to be displayed outwardly. As with Radha, it can be conveyed in a near-whisper. Whenever we have a true need, the thought of it is always in our minds. No matter what we are doing, we think, "If only I could have this," or "If only I could do that." That mental whisper is the real appeal of the heart. We are never so busy that we cannot whisper our devotion to God inwardly.

"His love is deeper still."

Following their arrest, Corrie and Betsie ten Boom were transported to the German concentration camp at Ravensbruck, a women's extermination camp notorious even in Holland. What became increasingly clear to them was the true spiritual reason they were there. From morning until lights out, whenever they were not in the ranks for roll call, Betsie always spoke to the other women about God's love for them. Even when she was near death, and so weak that Corrie had to bend close to make out her words, she continued to talk of their future ministry of love:

> [We] must tell people what we have learned here. We must tell them that there is no pit so deep that [His love] is not deeper still. They will listen to us, Corrie, because we have been here.

With devotion comes acceptance and attunement with the divine will. It has been well said that when we are really in love with God and in tune with the divine flow, we understand that things happen as they ought and that ultimately, everything works out for the best.

Attuning to the Infinite Consciousness: prayer

Along with meditation, prayer is a vitally important way to deepen one's attunement to the Infinite Consciousness. Although the Infinite Consciousness is beyond form, we can pray to that Consciousness in whatever form we choose (such as Krishna, Jesus, or the Divine Mother) and, from that form, receive answers and guidance.

"Give God your full attention."

Effective prayer, like effective meditation, depends on such qualities as will power and concentration. Speaking of the best way to pray, Paramhansa Yogananda gave the following advice: "Before praying, gain control over your thoughts and give God your full attention. You will see when you pray in that way that He answers marvelously! God answers all prayers, but restless prayers He answers only a little."

To pray effectively, Yogananda emphasized the following:
1) Pray to God, in whatever form you prefer: the Divine Mother, Jesus, Krishna, the Heavenly Father.
2) Pray with intensity and total concentration.
3) Pray from your heart, with devotion.
4) Pray with confidence that God is listening.
5) Be completely sincere with God, concealing nothing.
6) Pray believing, with utter faith that God will answer your prayer.

7) Pray with nonattachment. It is not wrong to ask God for material things provided you really need them, but even then leave it to God to decide what you should have.

Pray believing: "God is watching out for us."

In chapter 2 we discussed how, after the Taliban took effective control of Kabul (the capital of Afghanistan) in 1996, Kamila Sidiqi created a dressmaking business that eventually employed well over a hundred women. In order to help more people, Kamila later took on more expanded roles, including participation in a U.N.-sponsored program to train indigent women to make simple items like blankets and quilts that could be sold at the market. Kamila's new responsibilities exposed her to more dangers, including, on one occasion, being threatened with arrest at rifle point by a Taliban soldier.

Prayer, engaged in many times a day, was a vital part of Kamila's life. Explaining her refusal to abandon her efforts to help others, Kamila always affirmed her certainty that God would come to her aid:

God will help me because I am going to help my community. I put my life in the hands of Allah and I am sure he will keep me safe because this is work for his people.

Kamila prayed with the strong conviction (affirmation) that God would protect her. Kamila's practice of combining prayer with affirmation is an example of what Jesus Christ meant when he said we should "pray believing." By *affirming* that God would protect her, Kamila was not asking God to do everything for her. She was also putting her energy into the process. To "pray believing" renders the prayer itself more powerful.

After five years, on November 13, 2001, the Taliban abandoned Kabul. Kamila and her family survived.

A divine response to fervent prayer

Paramhansa Yogananda said that prayer is "talking to God," while meditation is "listening for His answer." There are times, however, when the dividing line between prayer and meditation blurs, when a person prays so deeply that he or she experiences, as one does in deep meditation, the inner presence of the Divine. Such was the experience of Kamala Silva, one of Paramhansa Yogananda's early disciples.

In her book *The Flawless Mirror*, Kamala Silva offers an inspiring account of her efforts to apply the power of prayer to an obstacle she describes as having the earmarks of a "seemingly unending karmic pattern." She poses this question: "How do we find within ourselves the strength to persist when our prayer efforts take on the weary desperation of a fruitless search for an answer?" Kamala was seeking to resolve a deeply troubling situation.

Despite feelings of desperation, Kamala believed, based on what she understood to be guidance from her guru, Paramhansa Yogananda, that prayer would bring the answer to her problem. She therefore appealed to the Divine "with fervent prayer." Three times God responded to her prayers by uplifting her into His presence. God's response brought deep and lasting feelings of peace, which Kamala realized was the solution to her problem:

> Nothing could disturb that Peace which lasted long enough each time to bring changes within myself. Often "answered prayer" comes in this manner. Problems are not always changed; we are.

Kamala's prayers were offered with such devotion, concentration, and intensity, that they became, in effect, a meditation. Each time she prayed, she was uplifted into an exalted state of communion with the Divine. The intensity of her prayers changed her in the same way that deep meditation changes the person meditating.

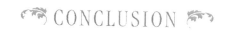

CONCLUSION

In seeking grace, also seek guidance.

Each individual aspect of magnetism is in itself magnetic—will power, concentration, kindness, solution consciousness. Working together they create a force of potentially tremendous power. Always remember, however, that material success itself—whether a new job, a compatible relationship, or increased income—is only a stepping-stone to perfection. From a spiritual point of view, every kind of success is potentially beneficial simply because the qualities that bring material success also bring spiritual success. Qualities that produce material failure also draw spiritual failure.

Wrong desires can also put the law of magnetism into operation. We see in the example of history's great dictators how selfish desires, backed by strong will power and concentration, can magnetize success and power, and cause suffering on a massive scale. We see also how their egoic self-seeking and callous indifference to the welfare of others created a negative magnetism, eventually leading to their downfall.

Whenever you are in need of grace, it is advisable to seek the guidance of the Infinite Consciousness. When your mind is calm, ask the Divine to direct you to the right course of action, and then act on the guidance you receive. The most effective prayer is to ask the Divine to guide you always so that you make the right choices. Toward that end, Yogananda recommended the following prayer:*"I will reason, I will will, and I will act, but guide Thou my reason, will, and activity to the right choice in everything."*

May your magnetism always be positive and uplifting, a blessing to your loved ones, your friends, and the world.

RESOURCES *for*
MEDITATION AND PRAYER

How to Meditate by Jyotish Novak: An easy-to-follow guidebook on the essentials of effective meditation. Crystal Clarity Publishers.

Affirmations for Self-Healing by Swami Kriyananda: Fifty-two affirmations and prayers to strengthen every aspect of your magnetism, including will power, positive attitudes, nonattachment, and attunement to the Divine. Crystal Clarity Publishers.

ABOUT THE AUTHOR

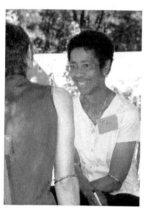

Naidhruva Rush was trained an attorney and has work in various legal positions i New York and California. Now liv ing at Ananda Village in Nevada City California, she serves as editor of *Clarity Magazine Online* and teaches classes on magnetism at the community's guest retreat: The Expanding Light. She is the editor of *In Divine Friendship*, co-editor of *Swami Kriyananda: A Life in God*, and co-author of *The Ananda Cookbook*.

Ananda's founder, Swami Kriyananda, writes that "magnetism is the most important thing in life." Naidhruva agrees: "An understanding of magnetism helps explain the seeming inequities of life. Through the lens of magnetism, everything falls into place."